Praise for *The Secret Power of Yoga*

"This sweetly voiced explication of the Yoga Sutras is disarming in its simplicity, charming and inviting the reader into the happiness of realizing that she/he is actually a manifestation of the Divine. I read it smiling all the way, and learning yoga philosophy as I was doing it."

—SYLVIA BOORSTEIN, author of *Pay Attention, for Goodness' Sake: The Buddhist Path of Kindness*

"Nischala Joy Devi has provided a dynamic new interpretation of the Yoga Sutras, one of the most important but esoteric guidebooks to deeper Yoga practice, that will make this wonderful ancient teaching accessible to modern readers and useful in their daily life. She has explained the essence of Yoga in a simple, direct, and relevant manner for all sincere students of the spiritual path."

—DAVID FRAWLEY (VAMADEVA SHASTRI), author of *Yoga and Ayurveda*

"Weaving together her deep knowledge of the Yoga Sutras with her many years of teaching and studying, Nischala Devi has created a very readable and insightful book. Her words ring with the authenticity of a committed practitioner, and the exercises she offers the reader can be truly life changing. But I must admit, I loved her funny and inspiring stories the best! A book to be read again and again."

—JUDITH HANSON LASATER, PH.D., P.T., yoga teacher since 1971 and author of six books, including *A Year of Living Your Yoga*

"Nischala Devi has given us a fresh and compelling new look into the mysteries of one of yoga's most important scriptures. Bravo! I heartily recommend her new book to all who want to understand (and trod) the practical path of liberation so brilliantly described by Sri Patanjali."

—STEPHEN COPE, author of *The Wisdom of Yoga: A Seeker's Guide to Extraordinary Living*

"This book has the feel of divinely guided inspiration. A loving call to every woman who walks the sacred journey. Nischala Joy Devi breathes new life, enthusiasm, creativity, and insights into the endless secret powers of yoga."

—LILIAS FOLAN, PBS host and author of *Lilias! Yoga Gets Better with Age*

"You hold within your hands a treasure box filled with priceless gems, collected by a most wise, gentle, and generous woman. This book promises to guide us, joyfully, to divine realization."

—SHARON GANNON, cocreator of the Jivamukti Yoga method

"Devi boldly reinterprets the Yoga Sutras of Patanjali from a personal acknowledgment of feminine intuition. Many women will find it refreshingly accessible and uniquely relevant to their spiritual quest on the Yogic path. Nischala brings a delightful emphasis on the celebratory Divine, inviting readers to allow this liberating text and the visualizations she's added, to illumine our own sacred journey to the heart."

—SARAH POWERS, international Yoga and mindfulness teacher

"A wise woman's guide to a life of peace and harmony. Full of heart and with a beautiful earthy wisdom, Nischala Joy Devi has crafted a whole new and feminine dimension to these ancient writings, bringing the age-old teachings of yoga right into our everyday actions and reactions."

—ANGELA FARMER, cofounder of Yoga from the Inner Body

"This book is revolutionary! With great skill, Nischala Devi guides us on a journey through the Yoga Sutras; not through a dry, intellectual dissection of words, but by bringing us out of our heads and into our hearts, where the intuitive insights of these teachings reside. An inspiring guide that will nourish your practice and your life."

—JANICE GATES, author of *Yogini: The Power of Women in Yoga*

"By 'telling the story in another way' Nischala Joy Devi allows these ancient Sutras from the soul to resonate in your heart. She delivers a bounty of stories, examples, experiential exercises, and new ways to awaken sacredness and experience life as a living joy. Like a green coconut, *The Secret Power of Yoga* invites you to hold it in your hands and open it. Read each Sutra aloud; through Nischala Joy Devi's tender and subtle rendering may you find every line fresh, fragrant, and deeply satisfying."

—SHANTI SHANTI KAUR KHALSA, PH.D., director of the Guru Ram Das
    Center for Medicine & Humanology

"Nischala Joy Devi illuminates a practical way to apply the Yoga Sutras to everyday living and spiritual awakening. Within the flow of her message is the trinity of *bhakti, jnana,* and karma. With *bhakti,* her approach and understanding come from the heart as she inquires into the heart of the matter. *Jnana* comes from her years of devotion to yoga. She complements this experience with cross-references to various classic scriptures. Karma is reflected at the completion of each sutra with a lesson that welcomes self-inquiry and calls for positive action. Nischala Joy Devi's commentaries, inspired from the feminine voice, will nurture many on the path of yoga."

—KALI RAY (SWAMINI KALIJI), internationally renowned yogini and
    founder of TriYoga®

The
SECRET
POWER
of
YOGA

A Woman's Guide to the
Heart and Spirit of the Yoga Sutras

NISCHALA JOY DEVI

THREE RIVERS PRESS
NEW YORK

ALSO BY NISCHALA JOY DEVI

The Healing Path of Yoga

Library of Congress Cataloging-in-Publication Data

Devi, Nischala Joy.
The secret power of yoga : a woman's guide to the heart
and spirit of the yoga sutra / Nischala Joy Devi.—1st ed.
1. Hatha yoga. 2. Exercise for women. I. Title.
RA781.7D4854   2007
613.7'046—dc22   2006026162

ISBN 978-0-307-33969-0

Printed in the United States of America

Design by Jo Anne Metsch

20   19   18   17   16   15   14   13   12

First Edition

To all the future generations of women and men

who will never even wonder if the

scriptures are also for women.

CONTENTS

Contents   ix

THE WISE WOMAN'S STONE

A wise woman, who was traveling in the mountains, found a
  precious stone in a stream.
She reverently placed the gem in her bag.
The next day, she met another traveler, who was hungry.
The wise woman opened her bag to share her food. The hungry
  traveler saw the precious stone in the wise woman's bag,
  admired it, and asked the wise woman to give it to him.
The wise woman did so without hesitation.
The traveler left, rejoicing in his good fortune.
He knew the jewel was worth enough to give him security for
  the rest of his life.
But a few days later he came back, searching for the wise
  woman.
When he found her, he returned the stone and said,
  "I have been thinking. I know how valuable the stone is, but
  I would like to exchange it in the hope that you can give me
  something much more precious. If you can, teach me the
  secrets about the power you have within you, the power that
  enabled you to, without hesitation, give me this precious
  stone."

A FOUNDATION
FOR TRANSFORMATION

TODAY, AN ESTIMATED 18 million people practice the physical aspect of Yoga. Most of them are women. Why is this? Is it because we've read in magazines that Yoga will give us a better body, tighter abs, buns of steel, or that we'll look and stay younger? Or perhaps we come to Yoga with problems we need fixed: physical issues, like stiff necks or sore backs, or emotional ones, such as depression, insomnia, or anxiety.

If these are the reasons we initially attend class, what keeps us coming back to Yoga, even after our problems are resolved or we've gotten in shape? Does something happen deep within us after we have stretched and squeezed and twisted and bent? Is there a special feeling that comes when we let go for just a moment and experience something magical inside? Something that seems familiar, something we have longed for or forgotten? Perhaps touching that mysterious part of ourselves is so powerful that we're motivated to return to it again and again.

"The journey of a thousand miles begins with a single step," said the Chinese sage Lao-tzu. Now, for growing numbers of harried Americans, a single step into a Yoga class begins a transformative journey into the vast world that unites body, mind, and spirit. The physical part of Yoga practice has become a gateway to this ancient spiritual discipline. Once we cross that threshold, we open ourselves to limitless possibilities, and to realms many of us have yet to dream of. When we let go and look within, the power we experience can transform our lives.

The Secret Power of Yoga is the knowledge that lies on the other side of that threshold, the knowledge that we are not just our bodies, our minds, or our emotions. The *secret* that brings endless *power* is *knowing that we are Divine Beings*. This knowledge can permeate our entire lives, bathing us in peace, joy, and love.

MORE THAN THE BODY

In the late 1970s, I was honored by an invitation to teach Yoga at a senior center. After teaching a class for the staff and answering their many questions, I was offered a job conducting a series of classes for the seniors themselves. My employment contract specified that I was not to do anything "spiritual" in the class, perhaps to keep anyone with strongly held religious beliefs from being offended. But how could I possibly teach Yoga and not be spiritual? Yoga's very essence is spiritual; it leads us back to our spirit. Yet the contract stipulated that I could teach only physical postures, breathing, and relaxation techniques. Chanting, prayer, philosophy, and meditation were not permitted.

I decided this was a challenge I would take on, so I signed the contract and began to teach class. I found myself holding back in the first couple of sessions. Then, after a while, the flow came more easily. During the deep relaxation, I could feel the peace inside myself and in the room. I felt satisfied.

About four weeks into the course, I arrived in the classroom to find several of the seniors huddled together waiting for me. "There she is! Come over here, we want to speak with you." A bit nervous and tickled at the same time, I walked over to the group.

"We want to know what *you* do when you practice Yoga," demanded one of the women. "We know there's more than what you're teaching us! You didn't get that peaceful from just stretching and breathing."

"Well . . ." I hesitated.

"Come on, tell us," they insisted. "What is Yoga *really* about?"

"My contract doesn't allow me to talk about the spiritual aspects of Yoga, and to me *that* is what it's about."

"We don't care what the contract says! Tell us more," they clamored.

So I did. They were delighted, and the class grew much deeper. Many of the people who had not been able to do the physical postures were able to experience inner peace through more subtle Yoga practices, an experience that they might otherwise have been denied. This was a great lesson for me about secrets *and* power. It seems that the real *power* of Yoga has been kept a *secret* for too long.

THE FEMININE FACE OF THE DIVINE

I'll never forget the opening scene from the movie *Yentl,* a tribute to women and their spiritual aspiration, directed by and starring Barbra Streisand. The narration begins with the line, "In a time when the story belonged only to the men . . ." Then we see a young, beautiful woman perusing the stalls of an open-air market in early-twentieth-century Poland. A lover of books and a clandestine scholar of the Holy Scriptures, she is attracted by a bookseller calling out to passersby, "Sacred books for men, storybooks for women. Sacred books for men, picture books for women."

She sneaks around to the men's side, where the sacred books are sold. "You're in the wrong place, Missy. Sacred books are for men," the bookseller tells her smugly. "Is it written that women cannot read sacred books?" she asks, with a slightly rebellious tone. Condescendingly, he replies, "Do yourself a favor and buy a picture book. Women like novels." Realizing that she has no other recourse, she says, "What if I say it is for my father?" "Why did you not say so in the beginning?" asks the bookseller as he takes her money and gives her the book.

This story has always touched me deeply. As a woman who has taught Yoga for more than thirty years, I have felt a great deal of frustration, and, at times, sadness, at the fact that virtually all aspects of Yoga—from translations of sacred texts to instructions on performing postures—have been interpreted almost entirely by and for men.

I feel passionately that it is time for women to explore and validate the experiences they feel deep within, experiences that men could never articulate for them. We need to know that what we are experiencing is not unusual or odd, but our true, unique, Divine nature shining through. This knowledge must then be passed on to everyone, both women and men, empowering all of humanity with its gift.

As *Yentl*'s story illustrates, it was not so long ago that women were not even allowed to read spiritual books, let alone provide commentary on them. Such prohibitions still exist in some cultures; women are forbidden to pray alongside men in many churches, mosques, and temples. Many religions draw strict lines between the sexes, laying out separate sets of commandments for women and men. Women may not be allowed to touch the holy books or even be in their presence. Those of us granted the privilege of reading the Holy Scriptures may notice that even in the great epics of thousands of pages, women are obviously absent in the text.

These traditions are so ingrained in our various cultures that we are often unaware of the patriarchal slant of doctrine and its consistent exclusion of women. The world has too long been viewed solely through male eyes. It is time for women to speak out and reinterpret the male-dominated scriptures in a way that resonates with our experience. And given the predominance of women practicing the physical aspect of Yoga, it seems natural to start with a woman's guide to the heart and spirit of the *Yoga Sutras*.

EXTRAORDINARY POWERS IN ORDINARY WOMEN

Among the hundreds of translations of the *Yoga Sutras* that exist today, almost all are written by men. Perhaps this is why so many of my female students have told me, "I have tried to read them, but they don't seem to relate to me. So I gave up. Can you recommend a translation that I can relate to?"

Until now, my answer had been "No," because I, too, have found most translations unsatisfying or inaccessible. Yet it was not an easy decision to interpret the *Yoga Sutras* from my own experience and from a feminine perspective. I knew I would face controversy and disapproval. After all, as many have told me along the way, I'm not a Sanskrit scholar, a professor, or even an intellectual.

Yet our story as women is filled with seers, healers, and visionaries who formed an integral part of society; most of them were not scholars or intellectuals. They were mostly unassuming people, living ordinary lives while exhibiting extraordinary powers. Their wisdom was derived from their very humility and open-mindedness. Very often, these women were tapping into their intuitive powers to heal or make awe-inspiring prophecies. Simple women reached into other dimensions as easily as stirring the soup or rocking the cradle, and in so doing they helped heal the sick and avert calamities.

Having this gift, this access to a higher order, was considered special but not unusual. These powers were once touted as "natural," something that all women could tap into. When viewed with an elevated consciousness, intuition was honored, not feared.

Tragically, this great and benevolent gift came to inspire fear. Women's intuition came to be regarded as "irrational," and women became second-class citizens. And in the darkest times many of the women exhibiting their intuitive powers suffered greatly at the hands of the ignorant. In the sixteenth and seventeenth centuries, countless women were tortured and burned alive as "witches," mostly in Europe and the United States. During these terrible times, most of those accused of having supernatural powers (which was often nothing more than the "power" of being beautiful) were women. Witch-hunting *was* woman hunting.

Thankfully, most women in modern society are not treated as harshly as we once were, but prejudices still remain. We are tempted to hide our gifts for fear of physical, mental, or spiritual persecution. But the great stories of women tell us that concealing our power is detrimental to future generations. Truly and joyfully embracing our power honors the blessed gift it was meant to be.

LANGUAGE OF THE HEART

The word *sutra* is related to the English word "suture," a thread that strings or sews things together. The *Yoga Sutras* weave together the warp and weft of our material and spiritual lives, creating an inspiring tapestry.

What many of us find lacking in the *Yoga Sutras* lies in their translations, written by and for male scholars from a left-brained, analytical perspective, often obliterating the wisdom they attempt to convey. It is my hope with this book to provide a unique commentary on the *Yoga Sutras* that emanates from the heart—an intuitive, feminine approach. Instead of translating the ancient Sanskrit to modern English, *The Secret Power of Yoga* reforms a variety of previous translations and interprets them in a new light, using "English of the heart" rather than the more conventional offerings that rely on "English of the mind."

Whenever a translation is offered, many of the prevailing prejudices, customs, and social standards of the time in which it was originally written are sifted into the mix. Since for a long time women were not highly regarded in a spiritual sense, the absence of emotionally centered parables, examples, and heart-centered teachings can be understood. The hundreds of commentaries and translations of the *sutras* written by men only further the exclusion of women in the spiritual world. Studies have shown that when the pronouns "he" or "him" are written or spoken, people do not make the leap of recognition that this also includes "she" and "her." This is why we see a movement in contemporary writing toward alternating "she" and "he," and in some cases, using s/he.

In addition, our modern culture tends to separate and even polarize the heart and the head, feelings and thoughts. Feelings are often considered inappropriate, wrong, or even scary. Yet if we look closely at the teachings of many ancient cultures, they describe the heart, not the head—embracing both thoughts *and* feelings. To deny feelings and validate only thoughts denies the very essence of our being. For this reason, I have chosen to use the terms "consciousness" and "heart," where the customary translation would read "mind" and "thoughts."

In Hindi the word "translation" means "telling the story in another way." *The Secret Power of Yoga* does precisely that, conveying the meaning of Yoga's most sacred teachings from a heart-centered, feminine view.

DIFFERENT AGES FOR DIFFERENT CONSCIOUSNESSES

During ancient times, when the great spiritual scriptures were being formulated, the world was open to many kinds of interpretation. According to historical accounts, many early civilizations divided time according to eras of human development. Plato, the great Greek philosopher, described a cycle of 24,000 years called the Great Year, during which the consciousness of human society expands and diminishes according to certain cycles. In yogic philosophy, the same idea comes forth as four *yugas*, sequential time periods of civilization similar in concept to Plato's Great Year.

THE FOUR YUGAS

The *Sat Yuga,* or the Golden Age, was the first manifested era. In this time people's behavior reflected their pure consciousness and integrated it smoothly with their humanity. Righteousness was eternal. One's duty to be true to one's spiritual nature was foremost. There was no competition, disease, depression, or struggle. Fruits of the earth and heavens were obtained by imagining, by being openhearted, and according to personal necessity. This could also be considered a more inclusive, feminine way of being. It sounds like the Utopian society that many of us dream about.

It was during this *Sat Yuga* that the *Vedas* were formulated. These great gems of wisdom were universal truths without reference to gender. They clearly proclaimed *we are one.* And from the *Sat Yuga* of evolved consciousness came the next three *yugas: Treta,* or the Silver Age; *Dvapara,* the Bronze Age; and *Kali,* the Iron Age. In each successive age, virtue was further obscured and righteousness increasingly faltered.

Many believe we are now in or emerging from the *Kali Yuga,* the nadir of enlightenment, and there is plenty of evidence for that claim. Egocentric thinking, greed, and fear have become the norm. Our respect for Mother Earth and for feminine values has declined, contributing to an epidemic of anxiety, depression, and hopelessness about the future. Most of us consider it a luxury to take time to retreat from the outer world to the realm of the spirit, and it is promoted as a blessing for the chosen few. With all this comes a devaluation of love, faith, and other spiritual virtues, causing them to hide deep within our hearts. We place little value on spiritual qualities; instead, we worship the material.

The good news is that we proceed through the yugas in a circular progression. So if we are now emerging from the Iron Age, the *Kali Yuga,* we are coming back around, toward the *Sat Yuga.* Because it has been many thousands of years since the time of elevated consciousness, little of that refined consciousness remains. But each of us holds some Golden Age consciousness within us, and it is ripening right now. The more we begin to acknowledge our inner spirituality and let it shine, the more we let heart and spirit reign supreme, the sooner we can make the Golden Age a reality.

UNLOCKING THE MYSTERY

The yogic path is the way to attain Golden Age consciousness. The *Yoga Sutras,* a great spiritual text and guide, embodies the purity of this *dharma* (righteous path). It weaves together a beautiful tapestry of essential wisdom and insights that allow us to know our Divine nature. Much of this wisdom is distilled and simplified from earlier sacred texts: the *Vedas,* the *Upanishads,* the *Bhagavad-Gita,* and perhaps some Buddhist texts. The *Yoga Sutras* uses the insights of these scriptures to depict the nature of consciousness and the path to liberation.

Though there is some uncertainty surrounding the origins of the 196 aphorisms in the text of the *Yoga Sutras,* historians have deduced that the *sutras* were originally compiled and codified by the great sage Sri Patanjali. It is thought that he lived at least 2,500 years ago. His aspiration (much like that of this book) was to restate these great teachings in a way that made them relevant to the people of his time. He also realized that if more people learned these great gems of wisdom, there was a greater likelihood that the essence of the teachings would be preserved and flourish.

The *Yoga Sutras* were transmitted orally, and without commentary, for a time before they were written down. When they were finally recorded in writing, they, like most other sacred texts, were engraved on leaves, and then sprinkled with a colored powder so that the letters or characters could be read. The leaves were stacked rather than bound so that the teachings could be easily

rearranged. The fixed arrangement in which we now most frequently see the *Yoga Sutras* is based on tradition.

The *Secret Power of Yoga* keeps the traditional format of most
translated texts of the *Yoga Sutras*. It has the four books, or *Padas*,
represented in their usual sequence and abides by the standard
numbering. This allows for easy study and the ability to compare a
variety of commentaries. Same or similar ideas are repeated in different parts of the text to help reinforce the importance of key
teachings. This repetition is common in other great teachings as
well, including the *Bhagavad-Gita* and the Old and New Testaments of the Bible.

The adaptations I have implemented are the creation of chapters,
summaries of certain sutras, and new commentary on selected
sutras. For example, most of the sutras in Book I, "*Samadhi Pada*:
Union with the Divine Self," and Book II, "*Sadhana Pada*: Cultivation of Spiritual Practice," as well as the first five sutras in Book III,
"*Vibhuti Pada*: The Divine Manifestation of Power," have full or
complete commentary. The remaining sutras in Book III and all of
Book IV, "*Kaivalya Pada*: Supreme Liberation," are summarized in
lieu of individual explanation.

The decision to comment on some sutras and summarize others
was made for several reasons. Books I and II are by tradition the most
widely expounded upon. Following that precedent, I have chosen to
go into some detail in those books, giving examples and suggesting
experiences or practices. The commentary extends into the first five
sutras in Book III, as they are part of the family of *Asthaanga Yoga*
("The Eight-Faceted Path") in Book II. Their appearance in Book III
is explained in the preface of the actual commentary, highlighting
their importance in understanding the whole of *Asthaangha Yoga*.

Books III and IV contain the most esoteric of the *Yoga Sutras* and
tend to be less accessible as the basis of a spiritual quest. This is
not to suggest that these books are insignificant; on the contrary,
they are offered in the *Yoga Sutras* to deepen awareness and

quench our thirst for the spiritual quest while continuing to reveal the essence of our true nature. They are best understood and realized when the concepts explained in Books I and II of the *Yoga Sutras* are intimately and thoroughly absorbed.

Also, because of the more occult nature of these later sutras, a heart-centered perspective would not necessarily enhance their interpretation in the same way it does for the sutras in Books I and II. As the awareness and insights portrayed in Books I and II develop, Books III and IV will more naturally beckon to you. I encourage you to read the many translations of the *Yoga Sutras* available that include these vital sutras.

The creation of chapters happened as I was contemplating the presentation of this Sacred Text. It became apparent to me that many of the sutras were grouped together representing the familiar venerable paths of *Bhakti Yoga* (Devotion), *Karma Yoga* (Service), *Jnana Yoga* (Wisdom), *Hatha Yoga* (Physical), and other categories. The *Bhagavad-Gita* (one of the texts from which the wisdom in the *Yoga Sutras* was drawn) was the inspiration for presenting these aphorisms in chapters, as it, too, is presented in chapters.

The sutras that inspire us to relate to the Divine from the heart form the chapter on *Bhakti Yoga,* the Yoga of Devotion. Those that relate to the physical are in the chapter titled "*Hatha Yoga:* Harmonizing Body, Breath, and Senses," and so on. I think it's a more manageable way to study the sutras, rather than the usual form of a long continuous column; a smaller group of sutras can be studied and assimilated with relative ease. Also, this presentation suggests a variety of ways to interpret the repeated sutras, offering a different angle in each chapter. This system conforms to the traditional numbering system found in the *Yoga Sutras*.

The sutras themselves were written as partial sentences and sometimes seem to be thoughts or feelings hanging in the air. It is as if they were jotted down in note form, reminding the teacher what to say next. The *Yoga Sutras* as they were written allow us to question and interpret them, and relate them to our particular situation and life. The eloquent pearls of wisdom are strung together to form one of the most concise, elegant, and complete teachings of Yoga available today.

Scholars and pundits East and West have translated and retranslated the *Yoga Sutras,* but most of the original translations from Sanskrit to English were done by a few Western scholars living in British-ruled India. Their hope was to shed some light on these great threads of wisdom as they made them available to the English-speaking population. These translators brought with them education, clarity, and experiences, along with their prejudices and cultural differences.

Western religious traditions vary from Eastern traditions in numerous ways. The fundamental understanding of Eastern wisdom is that divinity is granted by birth, whereas in the Western traditions divinity is usually something to continually strive for, and only a select few realize it, through grace or by their own accomplishments.

The mysteriousness and oddness that Western translators observed in the Indian culture caused them to cling even more to their familiar philosophies. This lack of understanding of the culture greatly influenced their translations. It is difficult, even now, for the Western mind to understand the complexities and subtleties of an Eastern mind-heart. The puzzle piece that seems to be missing is that, in Indian society, the heart and feelings are fundamental to, not separate from, life. This basic concept is the essence of their sacred prayers and scriptures.

THE GOLDEN AGE OF LEARNING BY HEART

We have all had the experience of learning something by rote to pass a test. Often we call this learning by heart. How many of us can remember this material now? But that which is truly learned by heart is never forgotten. The Secret Power of the *Yoga Sutras* can be found not by intellectual reading or discourse alone, but by deeply meditating on each aphorism, imbibing the spiritual truths and bringing them to our everyday life.

This way of learning may seem an unusual practice for our modern times, yet it is how spiritual teachings have been transmitted in Eastern culture from ancient Vedic times to the present. This learning process has three parts: *Sravana* (listening), *Manaana* (reflecting), and *Nididhyasana* (experiencing). Often a teacher would recite a sutra without explanation or commentary. The student would then retreat to reflect on the "feeling" the sutra evoked, thereby uncovering its meaning. After some days, weeks, or months, the student would return to the teacher and a discussion of a deep and profound nature would occur. The students were literally taking the teachings to heart.

The Secret Power of Yoga is oriented in this way. First the sutra is presented for silent and verbal repetition: you are encouraged to *listen,* understand, and feel the sutra. The commentary that follows invites you to *reflect* the wisdom of the sutra, using stories, parables, and personal insights to further instill the heartfelt meaning. The all-important *experiencing,* which is usually absent from the more traditional *Yoga Sutra* texts, is then proposed so the essence of each sutra can be integrated into everyday life.

Thought and Feeling

Sanskrit, the language of the sutras, is particularly well suited to this heart-centered approach because it is a vibrational language, one in which words resonate through countless layers of meaning. When this powerful vibrational language is translated literally into a very logical and straightforward language like English, many of its subtleties may be lost. The strength of the English language lies in precise, concrete explanations. It is less powerful when describing the subtler realms, the unity of the feminine and the masculine, and especially the intuitive realm.

Before we begin to formulate a word or even a thought, a feeling is experienced that stems from a vibration. This vibration that triggers the feeling is then translated into a thought, a thought to a word, a word to writing—a complex process that happens in a heartbeat. When we read, the word is connected to a thought, which then traces back to a feeling or a sensation. It happens so quickly and often that we fail to notice that each thought is the outgrowth of a feeling.

We see this phenomenon echoed in the formation of our physical bodies; the heart forms much before the brain. The process begins with the joining of the egg and the sperm, then the process of replication produces undifferentiated cells. Within a few short weeks of embryonic development, the cells begin to differentiate, and with those first specialized cells a tiny heart is formed. This early formation of the heart allows us as new beings to be guided by the rhythm of the spirit, and it is from the heart that feelings are born, flowing through us into each cell.

The brain, thought to be the provider of thoughts, develops much later than the heart. The heart remains independent in its rhythm until near the time of birth, when the central nervous system takes over the regulation of the heart. From then on the heart is reliant on the brain, and subsequently feelings seem to combine with thoughts and become virtually undistinguishable.

Yet when we feel something deeply, our ability to convey our experience in words lessens. Enraptured by the beauty of a magnificent sunset, our thoughts are stilled. We may find ourselves explaining to others, "Words can't describe such a deep feeling." Given the extraordinary difficulty of putting transformational feelings or divinity into words, it's easy to understand why rational thinking became dominant. We then superimpose the organizational structure of the physical world onto the spiritual realm, for lack of an adequately delicate design. Trying to express the subtle in mundane terms, we are perplexed. For this reason the *Nididhyasana* (experiencing) aspect of the study of the sutras can be the most vital. By honoring our feelings and the intuitive places of our being, we create the deep union between the heart and the soul. We can then spark the remembrance of who we *really* are, not just mirror the physical reality.

"True spiritual success is never gained through mere reading of books."
                                                              —*Yoga-Shastra*

SPIRIT OF THE SUTRAS

For many years I've been a student of the *Yoga Sutras*. I've sought to understand them from a "rational" view. This striving relaxed as the "heart perspective" invited itself into my study. Embracing the *spirit* of the sutras, rather than their literal meaning, allows me to integrate the sacred teachings at a much deeper level. In a way, it is like bypassing the mind and going directly to the heart and the soul. This allowed me to "feel" the vibration of what is meant.

As I am not a Sanskrit scholar, I have included only the few key Sanskrit words from these ancient texts, those that are most familiar. If this kindles your interest for more of the original language, there are scores of books and a few great teachers on the subject. The way I have chosen to share these great teachings with you is to reach into my heart, feel what wisdom they are imparting, and share that with you.

In *The Secret Power of Yoga*, the negative words that are found in the English language in abundance have been excluded where possible in order to bring a more positive vision to this Sacred Text. This was a difficult task considering that the English language has the habit of taking a negative word and adding a "not" or "un" to it, expecting the opposite meaning to emerge. But in actuality, the mind continues to relate to the root word, and we miss the important concept. For instance, the great virtue of *Astheya* in the *Yoga Sutras* is typically translated as "nonstealing." Upon hearing this, the mind cannot help but focus on "stealing"—exactly what we've been told not to do! For an opposite effect to take place, the word or words must be reinterpreted from "what not to do" into "what to do." *Astheya*, then, could easily be understood in positive terms such as "honesty," "generosity," or "integrity." So, rather than implying that people steal and proposing they refrain from this action, this text will propose that they be generous and honest and live in integrity.

Similarly, the sutra on *Aparigraha* is generally translated as "non-greed" or "greedlessness." Telling someone not to be greedy is like telling her not to think of chocolate. Once the notion of chocolate is planted in the mind, it's very hard to dislodge. A more positive approach goes to the heart of *Aparigraha* and unveils the positive perspective as "awareness of abundance," so that sharing what you have and taking only what you need follow naturally.

This same concept is often seen when words from other languages are adapted. Their literal meaning gives way to what they imply. For example, when they are put together, the French words *chaise* (chair) and *longue* (long), come to mean more than a long chair. "I am going to sit in the chaise longue" implies that this type of chair affords comfort and relaxation. We may then adapt the spelling to more easily fit into English grammar, as we have with "lounge chair." Here the meaning of the word *longue* (lounge) changes from "long" to "relaxation," describing its *effect* rather than what it actually *is*.

OFFERING THIS WISDOM FROM THE HEART

As a young yogini, I was on my way back from coleading a weekend retreat when my mentor, the swami in charge, informed me he would be leaving the ashram permanently in two days! My response was total shock. Ignoring my reaction, he continued, "I am in the third week of an eight-week *Yoga Sutra* course."

"What will happen to the class?" I asked, naively. With a smile he reached into his briefcase, handed me a copy of Patanjali's *Yoga Sutras,* and said, "Start studying!"

The night of the first class I taught I was very nervous. What would people expect? What did *I* know about the sutras? What if I gave them incorrect information? At the time there were very few translations available in English. The preferred way to learn the sutras was from a living teacher, one who taught as well as lived the wisdom. Still very young, I did not feel I had spent enough time sitting at my master's feet, absorbing the sutras in my own life. Certainly I was not steeped enough to teach others.

What was I to do? I did the only thing I knew how to do: pray. I prayed and prayed and prayed again. With that sincerity, my heart opened and I experienced the inner wisdom of the *Sutras.* My sense of clarity was restored. I now understood that knowledge received from an open heart transforms intellectual understanding.

My hope is that what I have presented here is useful, understandable, and in keeping with the truths of the *Yoga Sutras.* If they resonate with how you feel, take the teachings into your heart and make them your own. Meditate on them; use them in your life. Most important, remember the feeling of empowerment, the knowing that all of us, women and men alike, no matter how we may appear or sometimes act, are *Divine Beings* in human form.

From my heart to yours, I hope you enjoy the journey to discovering *The Secret Power of Yoga.*

Nischala Joy Devi

The
SECRET
POWER
of
YOGA

A JOURNEY THROUGH
THE SUTRAS

*Seek not to learn the sutras,
instead seek to learn who is the one
who studies the scripture.*

In "A Journey Through the Sutras," each sutra presented is numbered and in sequential order according to the traditional form. They are commented on individually or in clusters that have similar intentions or that when joined together complete a significant idea. This same clustering may also be applied to the section on *experiencing* at the end of each commentary.

The format of the sutras that follows supports the three stages or ancient ways of imparting knowledge described earlier: *Sravana* (listening), *Manaana* (reflecting), and *Nididhyasana* (experiencing).

The first stage, *Sravana* (listening), is facilitated by saying the sutra aloud, without the commentary. This aspect of listening is so vital, it is presented in three different ways at various places in the text. The first place you will encounter *Sravana* is in the list of complementary sutras at the beginning of each chapter. When repeated aloud in sequence, the rhythm of the words leads us to an understanding greater than each one could elicit individually. It presents the chapter's wisdom at the level of vibration.

You then meet each sutra individually before the actual commentary. Because you will have recited them at the beginning of the chapter, you will already be familiar with them. Take a moment to draw in a deep breath and, with wholehearted awareness, repeat the sutra or sutras aloud as you *listen* to the great teaching reverberating through your body, mind, emotions, and spirit. The opportunity to repeat this ritual will appear frequently throughout the commentary of each sutra. Each time it does, stop and *listen* to what the sutra is telling you. Allow the wisdom to be imparted before going on. In this way you will access the deeper, more intuitive form of knowing.

Finally, the section titled "The Yoga Sutras Heartfully Expressed" allows the meaning and flow of all the sutras in Books I and II and the first five sutras in Book III to be understood. Reciting them as one continuum allows the essence of the sutras to be conveyed and discovered.

Manaana (reflecting) is the stage that elicits a response from both rational thoughts and heartfelt feelings. This is accomplished through the traditional wisdom, stories, parables, and personal insights found within the commentary of the sutras. The intention is to satisfy the great spectrum of wonder, revealing a fuller understanding. As much as possible, relate this section to your life and circumstances. It will spark your heart's desire for knowledge.

Nididhyasana (experiencing) assimilates the earnestness gained from *Sravana* with the understanding gained from *Manaana,* unfolding the timeless truth of each sacred gem. These practices derive from the practical essence of each sutra. They enrich our perception by bringing us closer to the truth, often bypassing the questioning and rational mind. The *experiencing* often outshines any reluctance to change our previous ways.

BOOK I.

SAMADHI PADA:

Union with the Divine Self

HUMBLE BEGINNINGS

With humility (an open heart and mind),
we embrace the sacred study of Yoga.

1.1 With humility (an open heart and mind), we embrace the sacred study of Yoga.

THIS simple beginning holds many truths. Often this very first sutra is read quickly or even disregarded, which is unfortunate since this sutra is placed first to set the tone. It is here to remind us that our study and spiritual path benefit most when they are paved generously with humility.

DEVELOPING AN OPEN HEART AND MIND

As students of life, we often need to look at where we have come from to see where we are going. I was always enthralled by the subway in Paris. At each station a giant board helps you find your way. A little arrow indicates where you are, and with the push of a button you select your destination. As the destination registers, voilà!, a path lights up the most efficient way to get there. Wouldn't it be wonderful if our life path were that clear and simple?

Our present position has been determined by the past—all those crossroads where we made decisions, each path we've taken that brought us to our life as it is. We might be able to understand how we got where we are, but what would it have been like if other options had been followed? Another choice could have radically changed the present. Perhaps we took the tried-and-true course because it seemed easiest, or safest; perhaps at the time, it just didn't seem like there was any alternative.

> "What you are is what you have been, what you will be is what you do now."
>
> —Lord Buddha

Occasionally we meet someone who took an uncharted route, one less established. What in her life led her to become a trailblazer? What inspired her to leave behind the beaten path? The found path may have brought great adventures or great peril. Most of us are content to know that our future will be spiced with a few obstacles and sprinkled with safe adventures. Very few of us want to risk our comfort.

Custom and tradition play a major part in shaping our lives. We are so embedded in them that unless we are repeatedly shown a different way, we tend to live out our days under their sway. "We always have yams for Christmas. Why do you want to change tradition this year and have mashed white potatoes?" This tendency toward inaction and stasis can be difficult to overcome. But being creative and trying something different can be exciting and can expand your horizons. If it is carried beyond what is understood, it can cause rejection. Not wanting to offend, we may choose to reject the "new" idea that might have brought us renewed happiness and expansion.

Most of us in modern societies are very blessed. We are literate and have books as resources. Sacred Texts can be downloaded from the Internet. But even though they are so easily accessible, it is important to have the same regard and reverence for these sacred teachings as in times before.

THREE *GUNAS* (ASPECTS OF NATURE), TEACHERS OF HUMILITY

As students of spirituality, our yearning for the truth varies in intensity. Some of us may fit in a few spiritual practices at our convenience; others may dedicate their entire lives to their spiritual unfolding. Born with certain tendencies called the *trigunas,* or three attributes of nature, we are part of nature and are perpetually influenced by her.

This wisdom is drawn from the *Chândogya Upanishad*. It explains that all of nature, people included, contains an uneven mixture of the three *gunas*. One of the characteristics is always dominant. (See more on the *gunas* in Sutra I. 16, page 50.)

Sattwa is best translated as a sense of balance. *Rajas* is reflected in activity and overactivity, taking things to the extreme, while *Tamas* is inactivity, or being withdrawn, and can lead to difficulty focusing and acting, or inertia. The world and everything in it constantly moves between these three states, varying from minute to minute, day to day. This can be seen in the growth of a flower: *Tamas* is the plant in seed form, and *Rajas* is the growth action needed to bring about fruition. Once it has bloomed fully, intense action decreases, giving way to being, and *Sattwa* is present in the pristine flower blossom.

It is not possible to move directly from *Tamas* to *Sattwa*, although they may appear the same from the outside. To go from *Tamas* (inactivity), movement, or *Rajas* (action), must be traversed. From that movement dynamic stillness comes, as *Sattwa* (balance).

At night, as the natural light wanes, we become more indrawn and quiet (*Tamas*). During the day, when the light is strong, we tend to be outward and active (*Rajas*). At the two moments when day and night blend delicately together, at dusk and at dawn, there is balance (*Sattwa*). This quality is the reason dawn and dusk are observed by many traditions as auspicious times for prayer and meditation, a time of special equanimity.

In South India, a beautiful custom honors these three aspects of nature. When approaching a spiritual teacher for the first time, a prospective student offers the teacher a whole green coconut. (There, green coconuts grow on trees, a whole version of the ones we find here in supermarkets.) For the offering to be meaningful, the tree must be climbed and the coconut cut down. Then, according to tradition, the student has the arduous task of removing the tough green husk with a machete. This is a vital process, analogous to preparing the student's mind and heart for the teachings, to remove resistance or qualities of *Tamas*.

This process exposes the inflexible and brittle nature of the nut's hard brown shell. It represents the *Rajasic* part of our ego that is strong and thinks it knows everything. The coconut is now humbly presented to the teacher, or guru—a fitting name that means "one who removes darkness or ignorance, so that we may see the light of truth." With discrimination and deep compassion, the guru breaks open the hard brown shell of the coconut. The lily-white inner sweetmeat is revealed, symbolizing our *Sattwic* nature.

With humility (an open heart and mind), we embrace the sacred study of Yoga.

EXPERIENCING THE DIVINE IN EVERYTHING

Sit quietly, and light a candle if you wish.

Begin to make a mental note of your daily activities. How much of your day do you spend on simple repetitive chores that do not feel immediately rewarding? Do you sometimes feel they are a waste of time?

Begin by focusing on one of these activities, such as making the bed each morning. How can that be transformed into a spiritual practice?

Can you savor the smooth feeling of the linens? Can you have fun plumping the pillows? Put in some happy vibrations and feelings, so that when you get into bed at night, you will have happy dreams and a deep sleep.

Next, you might turn to the routine of checking voice mail, answering calls, filing papers, paying bills, washing dishes, or picking up your children from school.

Notice how each aspect of your life can be inwardly transformed to bring you to a place of presence and joy. There we recognize that the Divine is omnipresent.

WE ARE *ALL* DIVINE

THE following sutras enlighten us as to who we really are and how we experience life when we are in that state of knowing. They also remind us that as our consciousness moves outward, we separate from our essential nature. It is this identification with our Divine Self that leads us to joy.

Yoga is the uniting of consciousness in the heart.

United in the heart, consciousness is steadied, then we abide in our true nature—joy.

At other times, we identify with the rays of consciousness, which fluctuate and encourage our perceived suffering.

1.2 *Yoga is the uniting of consciousness in the heart.*

Yogah Chitta Vritti Nirodahah is the Sanskrit transliteration of this
well-known sutra. Through this one sutra we are able to know the
true essence of Yoga.

Deep within our hearts, we abide as pure Divine Consciousness.
But with the material world pulling us every which way, our consciousness is drawn outward. As our knowledge of the Divine
Self slowly fades, it takes with it the understanding of our true
nature.

Chit is pure universal consciousness and *chitta* is the same
consciousness individually expressed. *Chit* is the ocean of consciousness, vast and unlimited. At birth each of us gathers a small
quantity of this vastness and encases it in the temple of our heart,
as *chitta,* individual consciousness. Held for many years, it remains
unchanged. Then, at the end of our life, it is released back into the
ocean of consciousness; the recognition of oneness causes the
chitta to instantaneously unite with the *chit.*

Many translations of the *Yoga Sutras* link this sutra to notions of
controlling one's mind and thoughts. Trying to gather and control
the multitude of thoughts and emotions with no knowledge of their
origin is a daunting idea and a very difficult task.

It seems to be a compromised way of explaining the concept of
consciousness to a culture that does not have roots in the belief
that we are *all* Divine.

Consciousness abides in the heart, not in the mind, as many
believe. But when we realize that it is the *heart* that is the holder of
our consciousness, reunion—once understood to be a difficult
task—seems more likely.

When this sutra is translated referencing only the mind, the
emphasis is on control, restraint, or some form of restriction. It
encourages students to be harsh with the consciousness. But the

heart responds more readily to tenderness, and gentle, caring treatment of your consciousness is the best way to liberate it.

Notice your hand gestures when you are speaking to someone about who you are. Gesturing to my heart when I say "I am Nischala Devi" reveals the truth: "I live right here in my heart."

Yoga is the uniting of consciousness in the heart.

YOGA WITH A CAPITAL "Y"

Today the word "Yoga" conjures up the image of some difficult or contorted pose. Once relegated to a few faraway ashrams or caves, it is now practiced in gyms, health clubs, and studios all over the Western world.

What is being taught under the name of Yoga is a minute part of this great tradition, a microscopic focus on the physical. Yoga in its completeness is a way of life that allows for total transformation. But the physical postures, or asanas, can serve as an introduction to this distinguished wisdom tradition. Asanas reintroduce us to our bodies. Once we become friends with the physical, going inward to the spiritual becomes easier. Yoga in its completeness is a way of life that allows for total transformation.

AND THE BODY LEADS US

My early experience with Yoga, just like that of most Yoga students today, was mainly physical. Not a very physical person by nature, I nonetheless endured all the stretching and bending, hoping to find something more.

I brought my search into yet another Yoga class, this time at the Integral Yoga Institute, in San Francisco. As soon as I walked in the door, I was struck by a photo of the teacher beaming at me, face aglow with love and compassion. Somewhere inside I knew that Sri Swami Satchidanandaji, whom I later discovered to be an exalted Yoga Master, was the teacher who would ignite my soul, guiding me on my inner journey back to my own spirit. Integral Yoga enabled me to balance body, mind, and emotions, reminding me that through opening my heart I could touch the depth of my soul. Yoga became one of the greatest blessings of my life.

Yoga takes us back to the beginning of our journey of becoming human; we spark the memory that we are first and always an aspect of the Divine. The physical body was created as a temple to house this Divine light.

One starry night our mother and father felt that spark and before long, the largest and smallest human cells, egg and sperm, were united. We were on our way to a physical birth; our temple was being built. Our mission, as we were already Divine by nature, was to integrate our divinity with our humanity. No striving for divinity, no original sin, only the recognition of our true nature.

Born helpless into the physical world, our tiny being is over-whelmed by sensory stimulation. Finding the confines of the human body excruciatingly restrictive, we spend most of the time traveling in the astral world, brought back to earth only when the body needs food or a soiled diaper replaced, or when we are called back by the love of others on earth.

As time goes on, we spend more time in the physical body, and the processes of thinking and feeling begin to mature and occupy more of our consciousness. When at last we fully settle into the body, the challenge is to remember that we are Divine, as well as human, beings.

This is the essence of this sutra: to remember that we are, and always will be, Divine Beings who have become divinely human. Divine Consciousness emanates from our hearts, infusing our bodies, minds, emotions, and our very lives.

Yoga is the uniting of consciousness in the heart.

When we are able to realize this truth, all the sutras that follow *Yogah Chitta Vritti Nirodahah* are unnecessary. For most of us, however, the study of *all* the sutras is a necessary reminder, as we are quick to forget who we *really* are. As we embrace each subsequent sutra, we hope to uncover that which is obscuring this truth and come closer to living by it.

When delving into Yoga, it is up to you to choose how you image yourself *and* others. It is important to remember that *you are not the only one who is Divine.* Everyone is the same as you, just housed in different containers, shapes, and temples, embracing the same essence. Your relationship with the Divine Consciousness deepens or lessens according to your observance and treatment of yourself *and* others. Divine Being *or* human being? Divine Being *and* human being? Your choice.

The more we cloak our divinity, the dimmer the spark becomes. If we choose to shape our lives according to the lesser amount of light, rather than the boundless amount of light from the source, this becomes the yardstick by which all our experiences are measured.

Yoga is the uniting of consciousness in the heart.

AS SERENE AS A MOUNTAIN LAKE

Imagine consciousness in all its purity as a clear mountain lake. Gazing into the lake, we can see the mirror image of the mountains that surround it. This pristine illumination mirrors our Divine nature. While all is still and calm, the mind and heart rest in their Divine nature, and we experience love and oneness for all.

A gentle wind blows across the lake, and the clear images become slightly wavy. The crystal clear reflection of the light is disturbed, yet the distorted image can still be seen. If the wind continues to strengthen, the reflection of the mountains is soon completely obliterated.

The wind represents our thoughts and emotions, at first gentle and then strengthening. As the wind increases, it stirs up the bottom of the lake, and the clarity of the reflection is replaced by muddy turbulence. It may happen occasionally at first; and then slowly, without our realizing it, it becomes more and more frequent. Eventually, our Divine nature is no longer being luminously reflected.

After some time this motion causes the shore to wash into the lake, forming sandbars. Our thoughts and feelings form these clusters of habitual patterns, tendencies, and potentialities called *Samskaras*. The *Samskaras* accrue by the constant churning of the thoughts and emotions. Whenever any thought or feeling encounters the wind, it is easily fed into one of these patterns. Then our habits and tendencies become set and the mountains disappear from view.

The pattern of habit, or *Samskara,* is difficult to change, as our consciousness is often unable to reconfigure the obvious. An unexpected change in circumstances can be missed, if we look only for the predicted course. Once the sandbars have developed, it takes a great wind of change to modify their shape.

Yoga is the uniting of consciousness in the heart.

The lotus flower has long been a symbol for the unfolding of spirituality. It is one of the most elegant illustrations of the meshing of our human and Divine natures.

The lotus seed is planted and grows in muddy waters, below the surface of the lake, far from the light. Though the light is murky and unclear, the flower blossoms by drawing energy from within. As the bud passes through the muddy waters, it lifts its face to the sunlight and finally emerges. Miraculously, not a trace of soil remains on the flower. It lives in the mud yet is unaffected by it. This is an example for us to be in the world but not be adversely affected by it. The lotus flower teaches us that no matter how muddied the waters of our consciousness may become, clarity can always emerge from our spirit if the Divine Light guides us—even if it is only one tiny lotus blossom at a time.

> "I looked in Temples, Churches, and Mosques. I found the Divine in my heart."
>
> —*Rumi*

Yogah Chitta Vritti Nirodahah.
Yoga is the uniting of consciousness in the heart.

EXPERIENCING THE DIVINE SPIRIT WITHIN

In a softly lit room, sit as close as comfortably possible to a mirror.

Take a few deep breaths in and let them out slowly.

Allow yourself to relax.

Take a moment to look at your own familiar face.

Allow thoughts to drift away. Bring the awareness to your eyes.

Keep your eyes soft as you gaze deeply into them.

At first you may feel uncomfortable. (We rarely, if ever, look ourselves in the eye.) But the eyes are the windows to the soul, so take a look into your own.

Continue to relax and soften the gaze.

Find yourself going deeper within until you get a glimpse of the Divine Light that is ever present.

Repeat either to yourself or aloud, "I am a Divine Being."

Start by doing this for one minute, and build to five minutes or more.

As you allow your eyes to close, be still and experience any feelings that surface.

What did you experience? Could you feel the depth of consciousness within?

Practice two times a day for one week and observe how your newfound feelings and thoughts influence the vision of your true nature and other people's as well.

Each time you pass a mirror or think of yourself in any way, reaffirm, "I am a Divine Being."

1.3 *United in the heart, consciousness is steadied, then we abide in our true nature—joy.*

When consciousness reunites and remains undisturbed, our true Divine nature is revealed as joy. The expression of this joy is infinite love, which encompasses and then transforms everything it touches. Everywhere we look, we see the reflection of our Divine and joyful nature.

Many of us have had a glimmer of this feeling when we are falling in love. Everything looks brighter; even gloomy days cannot dissuade us from our bliss. We radiate joy and greet the world with openness and clarity. People smile at us, mirroring this loving energy back to us. This then serves to remind us of who we truly are, and the glorious cycle continues.

Recently, I was in the midst of making some very complicated travel arrangements. My flight schedule was a particularly important missing piece, so I called the airlines. As usual, I was quickly put on hold while some dreadful Muzak filled my ear. Every so often a mechanical voice assured me that my call was very important to the company. As the minutes ticked away, I believed it less and less.

Finally, an agent came on the line. It was, I admit, a complicated flight arrangement, but the length of time it took him to do it did not match the job. I was losing my patience. Using the idle pen while I was awaiting the schedule details, I began to write "*Om Shanti,*" the peace mantra, to regain my calm. Periodically he would come back to let me know that he was "still working on it." I thanked him and went back to my meditative writing.

Quite a while later, he came back, very apologetic that it had taken so much longer than he had hoped (me too!). We *finally* finished the arrangements and I thanked him.

"I want to thank *you,*" he said.

"Why would you want to thank *me?*"

"This has been one of the worst days of my life. Ever since I came in this morning, each call I received got progressively more abusive. I know I'm not quick, but I try to do my work diligently. But people have just been so impatient today. At two minutes to five I was writing up my resignation. Something told me to take one more call. It was you. You were so kind and patient and, well, loving to me. Even though I was slow, you weren't harsh to me. I was able to remember that I'm a good worker. Because of your kindness, I have decided not to quit. I pray that I may have many more customers like you. And for the ones that are not, I pray to have your patience."

I was amazed. It was as if he felt the vibration of the "*Om Shanti*" mantra, which enabled me to be so patient. Love is the common thread that united us. When consciousness is united in the heart, the reality manifests, and we know that we are all one in joy and love.

United in the heart, consciousness is steadied, then we abide in our true nature—joy.

1.4 *At other times, we identify with the rays of consciousness, which fluctuate and encourage our perceived suffering.*

Identifying with murky thoughts and feelings is like looking in a distorted mirror or a muddied lake. Those unclear images are often reinforced by the outside world. When we identify with grumpy or angry thoughts, the mind beams them outward. Similar thoughts and similar people are attracted to us as if magnetically. When we feel sad or fearful, friends who feel the same may call us. After all, misery loves company!

As we come to understand that our nature is joy and love, perceived suffering is unable to take root. Realizing that we do not have to be bound by any one interpretation, we alter our mode of identification. We then recognize and relate to our highest consciousness.

Imagine yourself standing in front of an enormous structure, one so large that it does not appear to have any boundaries. It is adorned with so many images, sayings, and words that the vastness keeps you engrossed. Even if at times the writings and images are disturbing, you remain attentive. Finally glancing around for a moment, you spot a small opening, not much larger than your eye. You never imagined this structure had any kind of depth. Its surface seemed so complete and all-encompassing.

Pressing your forehead to the wall, you peer through the small opening and are instantly transported to another reality, an incredibly beautiful scene filled with radiant light and glorious color. The disturbing images and messages that seemed so real only moments ago evaporate, like rain touched by the sun's radiance as it emerges from the clouds. You are transported through the portal to a peaceful vision. Once you taste the joy of living in beauty and love, you no longer find anything captivating about suffering.

KISS THE OTHER CHEEK

I was in Dulles International Airport, accompanying Mataji Indra Devi, one of my beloved teachers (then ninety-five years young) to her departing flight. Since saying good-bye to her students was always a lengthy process, she was running a bit late, so we sped to security, tossing her carry-on bags onto the conveyor belt. As she was about to walk through the metal detector, Mataji turned around and walked the other way!

"Oh no, what's she up to now!" I thought, conscious of the seconds ticking away. Oblivious to the movement of time, she had spotted an obviously unhappy security guard, whom I had sped by without noticing. She headed back toward him. Fully five feet tall in shoes, Mataji planted herself directly in front of the towering six-foot-five-inch guard. Standing on tiptoes, she reached up and took hold of his necktie. Using both hands as if climbing a rope, she pulled him down so that they were face-to-face. Stunned, he did not resist. I was aghast. What would happen? Would she be arrested? Should I try to stop her?

Mataji let go of his necktie with one hand and placed the other behind his head, and then planted a big kiss right on his cheek, complete with a loud smacking sound. Releasing both his tie and him, she turned and walked away. The guard was reeling, a smile of amazement on his face. She then casually walked through the metal detector, and, addressing my obviously surprised look, shrugged and said, "He needed that." As if that explained everything!

We are missing much joy if we allow the world to dictate the direction of our thoughts and feelings. But when our heart guides the focus of our consciousness, love is ever present in our life.

At other times, we identify with the rays of consciousness, which fluctuate and encourage our perceived suffering.

EXPERIENCING YOUR TRUE NATURE AS LOVE

Find a quiet place to either sit or lie comfortably.

Take in a few life-affirming breaths, and let them out easily.

Gently bring the awareness to your heart center, the seat of consciousness.

Observe as the consciousness is drawn away from the heart, attracted by any discomfort in the body. It could be your leg or arm, or a cramp in the back or neck.

Gently gather the consciousness and draw it back to the heart.

Repeat silently or aloud, "Yoga is the uniting of consciousness in the heart. I abide in my own true nature—joy."

Again observe as consciousness is drawn from the heart, attracted this time by the mind and its myriad thoughts.

Gently gather the consciousness and lovingly return it back to the heart.

Repeat silently or aloud, "Yoga is the uniting of consciousness in the heart. I abide in my own true nature—joy."

Observe the movement of consciousness from the heart toward emotions and feelings.

Gently gather the consciousness and lovingly return it back to your heart.

Repeat silently or aloud, "Yoga is the uniting of consciousness in the heart. I abide in my own true nature—joy."

Gently repeat this sutra any time you notice consciousness moving away from the heart. It will aid you in bringing it back to your heart.

Slowly take in a few deep breaths. Notice how joyful you feel, living from the heart.

It is helpful to practice this for at least ten minutes each day and to repeat frequently throughout the day the sutra "Yoga is the uniting of consciousness. I abide in my own true nature—joy."

RAYS OF CONSCIOUSNESS

CONSCIOUSNESS expands outward from the heart as we become part of the physical world. This cluster of sutras enables us to understand how consciousness ventures from its home in the heart and manifests as emotion and thought. The degree of clarity to which it manifests forms the framework for our life.

Dividing into five, these rays of consciousness polarize as pleasant or unpleasant.

The rays manifest as knowledge, misunderstanding, imagination, deep sleep, and memory.

Knowledge embraces personal experience, inference, and insights from the wise.

Misunderstanding comes when perception is unclear or tinted.

Imagination is kindled by hearing words, seeing images, or experiencing feelings.

Deep sleep allows us to withdraw from conscious awareness.

Memory is when a previous experience returns to conscious awareness.

1.5 *Dividing into five, these rays of consciousness polarize as pleasant or unpleasant.*

Our thoughts and feelings are trained by habit to flow in predictable patterns, which determine whether our life fosters a sense of ease and happiness or turns from it. These patterns are so ingrained that even the hint of a possible directional change is incomprehensible. Constant identification with these patterns forms our belief system, a blueprint for our lives.

Many belief systems seem to hold that difficulty is beneficial, and growth comes only with pain. This is reinforced by the all too popular adage "No pain, no gain."

Perhaps we should reconsider this philosophy. A small measure of discomfort *may* be necessary to encourage growth, but how much? Our hearts hold the hope that growth can be gained through love and kindness.

After a complicated dental procedure, I was given a prescription for pain medication. "Thank you," I said, returning the slip to the dentist. "I don't take any medication."

"You might want to rethink that. Research has determined that when even moderate pain is experienced, the healing process is inhibited," my dentist said, returning the prescription to me.

Could this same phenomenon be experienced on other levels, too? What if instead of hoping for pain to bring rewards, we simply turned directly to the rewards themselves? We may not have the ability to determine the outcome of every situation. We can, however, choose how it affects us, by looking at it from another view. Often I refer to those unpleasant times as the "cosmic itch," which presents just enough discomfort to keep me from getting too complacent yet not enough to cause real difficulty.

Whichever belief system you subscribe to, know that you possess the power to affect your life's patterns and dreams. When a thought, feeling, or situation arises, it will naturally flow into the groove that presents the path of least resistance. Which beliefs present that avenue for you?

Imagine if they were like those of a dear friend of mine. "How are you?" I asked her, on seeing her for the first time in a long while. "I am in my usual state of grace," she replied. "The difference is, this time *I know it!*"

We are all in a constant state of grace, yet how often do we remember?

Dividing into five, these rays of consciousness polarize as pleasant or unpleasant.

EXPERIENCING HOW YOUR BELIEF SYSTEM INFLUENCES YOUR LIFE

What is your belief system? Do you feel closer to the Divine when you are in crisis or in joy?

Do you invite hard times because you believe that they will help you to become stronger?

Notice how you have set up your life to foster those beliefs. Are you happy with your choice?

Pick one particular feeling, thought, or phrase that you use frequently. It could be "Life is hard" or "Life is good."

Actually count how many times you use it in a day. How does the meaning influence your day and ultimately your life?

Only you have the power to change your life.

1.6 *The rays manifest as knowledge, misunderstanding, imagination, deep sleep, and memory.*

When consciousness ventures from its center, it forms rays that take on diverse characteristics and intents. With clarity and a keen sense of observation, these rays can be understood as distinct aspects of the one consciousness.

The rays manifest as knowledge, misunderstanding, imagination, deep sleep, and memory.

1.7 *Knowledge embraces personal experience, inference, and insights from the wise.*

The first ray of consciousness is *knowledge,* which then divides into three distinct aspects. These three aspects of knowledge illuminate the other rays of consciousness.

CAN YOU RELY ON PERSONAL EXPERIENCE?

The first aspect of knowledge is personal experience. Where does this come from? The senses gather information from the sense organs, which are then interpreted by the mind and emotions.

When this information resonates with our bodies, minds, and emotions, a clear and identifiable knowing is confirmed. Living from that place, the whole universe seems to make sense. Knowledge becomes a steady, reliant friend.

But it is not always so amicable. If the mind and instruments of perception are murky, our perception becomes tainted or false. Our mind and senses can trick us. At the scene of an accident, for instance, if there are four witnesses, then there are at least that many versions of what happened. How could that be? It was the same event viewed by people with the same sense organs who saw it with their own eyes and heard it with their own ears.

The organs of the senses are not faulty; it is our individual perceptions that distort. As a scene is filtered through thoughts and feelings, past experiences and prejudices, it becomes different for each person. Until they shine with perfect clarity, take your personal experiences with an ounce of caution.

Knowledge embraces personal experience, inference,
and insights from the wise.

IDENTIFYING INFERENCE

The second aspect of knowledge is inference. Often we experience knowledge from a deep place that carries no apparent reasoning. We honor this as our intuition. It is a sense of knowing that may have no other explanation or experience to reinforce it. It stands in its own power.

Inference, however, based on lucid perceptions can also help us to discriminate and to make decisions.

Seeing a cow give milk, we may then infer that all cows give milk. We confidently believe that if we can find a cow, we'll find milk. Only with careful scrutiny can we observe the difference between a cow and a bull. Without discrimination, inference might encourage us to attempt to milk a bull, putting us in peril with not a drop of milk to be had.

This aspect of knowledge can be very precarious. Many prejudices perpetuated by inference are taken to be the truth. Hearing about an individual from a minority race, religion, or national origin who has committed a crime, many find a temptation to lump all people "like that" together as criminals. If someone in a fancy sports car cuts you off on the highway, you might find yourself thinking harsh thoughts about the wealthy.

Instead of these judgments, use your power of inference to give people the benefit of the positive. Making gross generalizations places people in opposition, and what we do to others, we do to ourselves. Look for the good in all things and all people. Hone your skills of discrimination and keep your heart open when you initiate inference. And always honor your intuition!

Knowledge embraces personal experience, inference, and insights from the wise.

RECOGNIZING THE WISE

This aspect allows us to acquire knowledge through the wisdom of others that is often based on their own deep understanding or experience.

For many, knowledge is legitimized when it is written or spoken by an expert or a prophet. We consult the Holy Books (Bible, *Koran, Vedas, Yoga Sutras, Gitas,* etc.). Traditionally forward-thinking scientists or intuitive clergy boldly analyzed and interpreted formulas or passages, often challenging their peers. When they were able to prove their theories as "correct," they became truth. We then embrace these "truths" as our touchstone. For some of us, therefore, knowledge must be accompanied by a deep resonance within.

At the time when the scriptures were formulated, very few common people were literate. Before the time of written scriptures, most of the teachings were orally transmitted, often to a congregation; for the especially devout, they were conveyed directly from teacher to student. When the direct transference of wisdom was accomplished, any doubts were alleviated. In those times of oral tradition, minds and emotions were sharper and less cluttered. The spoken word went deeply and directly to the heart.

As the scriptures were committed to writing, they underwent a continuous process of evolution, modification, revision, and translation. This was accomplished by a small group of men who were privileged enough to have a high level of education. Often segments were lost, truths omitted, and stories reinterpreted. It is often difficult for women to accept many of the scriptural concepts as truth because of their inherent prejudices against the sacred feminine. Miraculously, there are still a cherished few of these writings that ring out with a truth that resounds with women. It is up to us, however, to find the flowers among the weeds.

The greatest wisdom is the insights experienced in our own hearts. This is the wisdom we cannot deny. The more we trust and honor it, the more it guides us.

> "All truths are easy to understand once they are discovered;
> the point is to discover them."
>
> —*Galileo Galilei*

Knowledge embraces personal experience, inference, and insights from the wise.

EXPERIENCING THE THREE
WAYS OF KNOWLEDGE

Choose a concept or a passage from a great spiritual book. Or choose anything else that inspires you.

While reading, observe if it resonates with your heart. Do you feel harmonious with the basic concept? Are there some aspects of it that you resonate with more than others?

Search until you find a passage or a commentary that supports your feeling.

If one does not reach you precisely, reword, rearrange, or broaden the idea until you feel in accord. This allows the passage to be more inclusive and sing to your heart.

When you hear its song, you are experiencing true knowledge.

1.8 *Misunderstanding comes when perception is unclear or tinted.*

Misunderstanding, the second ray of consciousness, is a common fluctuation that may cause us a great deal of unpleasantness. Often we assume with certainty that our minds and emotions correctly interpret our sensory input, but do they? Many longtime resentments are perpetuated due to misunderstanding. Family members may hold grudges for years, and even take them to their graves. Often the next generation is unaware of the feelings of bitterness they inherited from their relatives.

Listen carefully with heart and mind, and ask for clarification when there is even the slightest doubt. And, most important, use a liberal amount of forgiveness for mistakes—after all, the mistake might be yours.

Misunderstanding comes when perception is unclear or tinted.

EXPERIENCING WAYS TO CLARIFY UNDERSTANDING

Recall a recent time when you were involved in a misunderstanding. It could have been important or trivial. Is it clear to you where the misunderstanding occurred?

> *Go through the whole scenario again from the beginning, and bring clarity where it was absent before. Try to smile at the way things were misconstrued. Imagine the outcome to be comfortable for all concerned.*
>
> *When there is a misunderstanding, can you forgive even if you were inconvenienced or put in an uncomfortable situation?*
>
> *Can you forgive even if you are right?*
>
> *Would you rather be right or happy?*

1.9 *Imagination is kindled by hearing words, seeing images, or experiencing feelings.*

Imagination is the third ray of consciousness. When it is illuminated, it becomes the path leading us to and from our heart's center.

Imagination allows us to create an unlimited number of both pleasant and unpleasant experiences. An image is felt, and from that a thought, a word, or an action sprouts. When it is bathed in negative imagination, the image can have an unsettling effect. For instance, worry is the most prevalent form of imagination for many people. And all of us have been frightened by something that appeared to be there only to later discover that it was not a threat to us or our loved ones. Do you easily reach for the worst-case scenario? When the imagination goes so far out, it takes immense effort to bring the mind and the emotions back to calm.

Perhaps taking a pleasant stroll to the mailbox, you find an unpleasant surprise: a letter from the IRS. Likely your whole body goes into a stress response, terrified that you are being audited or owe money. In an instant you are trying to figure out where you can borrow the money. The envelope is not even opened yet! Holding your breath, you open it—and an instant smile of happiness travels from your face to your whole body. It is a refund, and a big one at that! Worry and negative imagination led you to anticipate the worst.

Such an immediate and transforming reaction affecting the whole body is one of the reasons imagination and imagery have become very powerful tools for healing. A positive image can elevate us and support us to heal. The opposite can cause many physiological systems to malfunction and cause disease.

Imagination is kindled by hearing words, seeing images, or experiencing feelings.

TAKING THE TIME TO DAYDREAM

Daydreaming is another form of imagination. Although it is usually thought to be a waste of time, science is now finding that it actually provides a minivacation. I was always scolded in school for daydreaming and wasting time. Who would think that I now teach that very skill to people to help them heal! Every great individual—thinker, artist, musician, gardener, cook, mother, or anyone else—uses imagination as a way of setting the creative process in motion. What looks like a daydream is in fact your most productive moment. It is in your power to formulate pleasant *or* unpleasant experiences.

> "Imagination is greater than Intellect."
>
> —*Albert Einstein*

Imagination is kindled by hearing words, seeing images, or experiencing feelings.

EXPERIENCING YOUR CREATIVE, POSITIVE IMAGINATION

How keen is your imagination? Do you imagine the absolute best for yourself?

Write down your hopes and dreams as an affirmation to help solidify them on the physical plane.

Your imagination is infinite; use it lavishly to the smallest detail.

If you are experiencing a physical or emotional imbalance, use your imagination to create the affirmation that will allow you to see yourself whole and healthy.

Engage all of your senses as part of the affirmation. The more real it seems to you, the more likely it is to become real.

Each day recite and experience your affirmation as it enhances the new image you have created of yourself.

Practice this with any and all aspects of your life.

1.10 *Deep sleep allows us to withdraw from conscious awareness.*

Deep sleep allows us to withdraw from conscious awareness, offering us the luxury of temporarily forgetting. It is like having a holiday from thoughts, emotions, worries, and cares by completely letting go. Sleep is necessary for health and balance, providing a time for the body to repair itself and for the mind and emotions to release.

If we are to function effectively and lovingly during the waking hours, the deep sleep that allows us to rest in our inner consciousness is of prime importance. When we are well rested, our spiritual practices harmoniously unite all aspects of our being, allowing us to know who we really are.

> "That we are not much sicker and much madder than we are is due exclusively to that most blessed and blessing of all natural graces, sleep."
>
> —*Aldous Huxley*

Deep sleep allows us to withdraw from conscious awareness.

EXPERIENCING THE EFFECTS OF DEEP SLEEP

Can you observe the effects of a good night's sleep on your body? Your mind? Your emotions?

Notice how you feel after a deep, dreamless sleep. Refreshed and rejuvenated?

Notice how you feel after a fitful night of dreaming and waking. Tired, and perhaps a bit cranky?

Can you relate how you slept to what you watched, read, discussed, or ate the night before?

What was engaging your consciousness during that time of deep sleep? You may not be able to know exactly what happened during sleep to your body, mind, or emotions, but both the positive and injurious results can be felt.

Observe how your sleep pattern affects your life.

1.11 *Memory is when a previous experience returns to conscious awareness.*

All day long, year after year, we take in impressions, which are then filed and stored within us. We are actually made up of volumes of memories that then create our present and future. We choose which memories are kept ready and available in the forefront—and which are tucked away in the unconscious. Our concepts and ideas need to be carefully weeded and released on a regular basis so that our consciousness can keep evolving. Without this constant vigilance, we find we live with stored memories that anchor us in the past.

Repressing unpleasant memories, though, can lead to serious problems. Although dormant, unpleasant memories can be triggered at very inopportune moments, causing us to relive the discomfort they brought us. A word of casual conversation with a friend may conjure up a memory of betrayal or abuse. This triggers feelings from the past that come flooding back, overwhelming present emotions. Misplaced hurt or anger may encourage an argument. Later, when trying to understand what happened, you may realize that it had less to do with your friend than with a long-forgotten memory relived.

On the other side, if pleasant *memories* are deeply planted, they may have the ability to encourage an easeful feeling even if life's woes are ever present. A situation may present itself in which you would have felt uncomfortable or threatened, yet recalling the pleasant memory radiates a feeling of peace.

The yogic practices help us release memories without having to express them either outwardly or in dreams. They also help dissolve unwanted thoughts and feelings as they are forming, relieving the need to see them to fruition or preserve them for a later time.

Sometimes while sitting still in meditation or holding an asana (pose), a memory will escape from the bottom of the mental-emotional lake. Like a bubble, it will float through layers of the subconscious and then pop on the surface of the conscious mind. It then becomes your choice to keep it or let it go. By bringing it up at a time of peace and relaxation, you can control your memories, rather than letting them control you.

Memory is when a previous experience returns to conscious awareness.

EXPERIENCING THE RETURN OF MEMORIES

Bring a memory of your choosing back to consciousness.

Notice what kind of physical sensations and emotions come with it.

Are you able to separate the memory from the sensations? Or are they one and the same?

Try to find its origin inside your body.

Then, try gently to release the memory.

How does the experience of release feel?

PRACTICE AND REMEMBER

H ERE we are given the key to balance and the way of power that aids us in our quest for the True Self.

Consciousness is elevated by Abhyasa (Devoted Practice) and Vairagya (Remembering the Self).

Devoted Practice, Abhyasa, cultivates the unfolding of consciousness.

Abhyasa is nurtured by a sustained, steady rhythm and a dedicated heart.

With constant Remembrance of the Self, Vairagya, all yearnings fade.

When consciousness unites, it remains clear and unaffected by the external changes of nature, the gunas. This is the ultimate Vairagya.

By cultivation of Abhyasa and Vairagya, the intellect becomes keen, reasoning is clear, bliss is reflected to all, and outward identification unites with the Supreme Consciousness.

With continued awareness, we identify only with the pure consciousness residing in the heart.

Through identification with pure consciousness,
the physical world can be transcended.

This identification is enhanced by faith, dynamism,
intention, reflection, and perception.

To the dedicated and devoted, the Divine truth is revealed.

Spiritual Consciousness develops in direct proportion
to one's dedication.

1.12 *Consciousness is elevated by* Abhyasa *(Devoted Practice) and* Vairagya *(Remembering the Self).*

Here are two necessary components to reunite us with our True Self. Imagine that *Abhyasa* (Devoted Practice) and *Vairagya* (Remembering the Self) are two wings of the same bird. They are companions in play as they flap in unison enabling the bird to fly: when they are seemingly still, the bird glides. Moving into a change of position, one wing lowers and the other raises. This complementary movement allows the bird to fly with grace and ease. Rhythm is the secret to the bird retaining its elevation; for us, rhythm keeps our consciousness elevated.

When a devoted practice is cultivated, that inspires us to remember the Self. This balances and brings grace to our daily rhythm. As we remember the Self, the effects of our simplest actions are considered. We relinquish old mindless habits *(Samskaras)* by intentionally choosing what to invite into our bodies, minds, hearts, and lives. "If I eat this large meal late at night," you might ask yourself, "will I be able to wake up early and be alert for *Sadhana* [spiritual practice]?" The correlation between eating a big meal in the evening and feeling light and alert in the morning becomes clear.

It takes time and patience to cultivate such understanding. At first opting for immediate gratification, we may toss all consequences to the wind and indulge in that large meal at night. The lethargy of the next morning encourages us to have a deeper consideration the next time a similar situation presents itself. With this new awareness, we are able to evaluate both the immediate and long-term effects of our decisions.

In order to soar, the bird needs both wings to flap to the same rhythm. When in balance, both wings are strengthened. Whatever challenges are encountered, with *Abhyasa* and *Vairagya,* we embody the skill and assurance to ride the currents.

Consciousness is elevated by Abhyasa *(Devoted Practice) and*
Vairagya *(Remembering the Self).*

I.13 *Devoted Practice,* Abhyasa, *cultivates the unfolding of consciousness.*

To continually elevate consciousness, it is necessary to cultivate
Abhyasa—devoted spiritual practice. As we develop a deep friend-
ship with our inner Self, the fluctuations of thoughts and feelings
recede and the comfort of the truth unfolds. Our senses and the
material world constantly pull us outward, away from our inner
consciousness. With deepening devotion we are encouraged to
rediscover that Divine spark within. It then becomes our first
choice of identification in any given situation.

Devoted Practice, Abhyasa, *cultivates the unfolding of
consciousness.*

I.14 Abhyasa *is nurtured by a sustained, steady rhythm and a dedicated heart.*

Here we are given three ways to nourish and deepen a methodical
spiritual practice. What exactly is a devoted practice? What does it
mean to nurture our practice by a sustained, steady rhythm? And
for how long? A month? A year? Ten years? It is not possible to
have a formula to determine something as acutely personal to each
individual.

Often students will become frustrated. "I've been practicing
meditation now for three months and I still don't feel anything
different."

"What is it," I ask, "that you expect to feel?"

"I don't quite know, but I expected something otherworldly to happen," they answer.

Even if we do not realize it, what we are seeking is the sense of wholeness. This sense is so familiar that often we forget that it is always with us. The time we spend each day in communion with ourselves is such an integral part of our lives that when it is absent, we feel unbalanced and out of sorts. Rhythm of practice, on the other hand, can be one of the most stabilizing effects of our life.

The rhythm of a devoted practice is sustained and steady when you no longer have to ask "Should I sit for meditation today?" Now there is no need to make excuses, to look for a reason to take a day off. A Benedictine monk who devoted himself to spiritual practices for more than thirty years once told me that if for one moment he hesitated or questioned, he would have left his vocation. Observing his deep inward smile, it was obvious what he would have missed.

Abhyasa *is nurtured by a sustained, steady rhythm and a dedicated heart.*

WHOLEHEARTED DEDICATION DEVELOPS A WHOLE HEART

In order to sustain a dedicated heart, choose a practice that encompasses the richness of spirit in everyday life, one that nourishes you on all levels. If you are devotional by nature, tend toward chanting or other practices that complement the heart-centered feeling. If you are more intellectual by nature, you might be attracted to the study of Holy Scriptures. The predominantly physical person might enjoy the more active asanas (poses). But for the most harmonious effect, try to create a well-rounded balance in your choice of practices.

Simple repetition is not enough for true *Abhyasa*. Our practice may be as steady as a drumbeat, yet to fully embrace the spirit of the activity, a deepening must take place. A metronome beats a steady rhythm, but it is the heart of the musician that imbues the music with spirit and life. This kind of transformation takes place when our practices, traditions, and teachers are wholeheartedly honored.

In time most daily rituals—cooking, driving, eating, giving someone a kiss good-bye, even meditating or engaging in spiritual practice—can become rote or routine. Keeping the enthusiasm alive is the key. After months or years of doing the same poses, breathing techniques, and chants, the heart may lose its hold on the practice. Don't discard them; instead, rededicate your heart to them. Lavished with love, they can be transformed into a practice that resonates for you. The striving then stops as the heart takes over. The ordinary is transformed into the extraordinary!

> "The secret of genius is to carry the spirit of the child into old age, which means never losing your enthusiasm."
>
> —*Aldous Huxley*

Abhyasa *is nurtured by a sustained, steady rhythm and a dedicated heart.*

EXPERIENCING THE RHYTHM OF YOUR SPIRITUAL PRACTICE

What is the rhythm of your practice?

Is it steady like a metronome?

Is the rhythm too fast or too slow? Regular or irregular?

Is there anything you can add to enhance your heart's participation in the practice?

Introduce flowers, a plant, a beautiful mat, a pillow, or a photo of nature or of an exhalted being into your sacred place.

Do whatever you can to encourage the union with the Divine Self.

1.15 *With constant Remembrance of the Self,* Vairagya, *all yearnings fade.*

As our focus turns toward "Remembering the True Self," we naturally identify less and less with external desires or wants. This perspective reveals that we are merely the temporary caretakers of whatever we possess. With this attitude, nothing binds us. As life bestows gifts upon us, we are delighted. With their revocation, we may feel momentarily upset, but with the grace of remembering our Divine Self, our emotional equilibrium is quickly restored.

Through Remembering the Self, or *Vairagya*, we become lucid and vibrant like a diamond. Millions of years of pressure on a simple lump of solid coal transforms it into a pure, transparent diamond that reflects and refracts light. This prismatic effect showers rainbows of colors on everything without discrimination *(viveka)*. The diamond also appears to take the color of any object nearby. But once removed, it is perfectly colorless again. Likewise, when our minds and hearts clearly reflect our true nature, we may acquire many things, but nothing permanently taints our clarity.

With this lucidity, we enthusiastically adopt that which enhances the light, and redirect that which dims it. As we become free, we become more and more comfortable with the natural flow of material things. Much of what we yearn for comes to us. We enjoy the treasures of the world while they are with us, knowing full well we will not bind to them, nor they to us. And as they depart, our arms open wide and let them fly. Steady in both circumstances, we remember who we really are.

This concept has its greatest challenge when we are separated from our friends and loved ones, especially without our permission or when it seems permanent. Our heart feels a vast emptiness where it was once filled with love. At these times it takes great strength to restore and sustain our equilibrium. By securing a place within our hearts to hold their love and by continuing our devoted practice, our balance is more easily reestablished.

With constant Remembrance of the Self, Vairagya, *all yearnings fade.*

CAN WE BE ATTACHED TO NONATTACHMENT?

Often *Vairagya* is explained as "nonattachment." This is a harsh misunderstanding, which promotes avoidance of a situation or a person, based on translations that guide us toward what not to do, instead of what to do. This interpretation of *Vairagya* grants permission to be cold and uncaring, "nonattached," as a way of not getting hurt by others, or negatively attached. Such a stance is often accompanied by a large dose of fear and insecurity. It is exactly the opposite of the oneness our hearts are leading us to.

Similarly, we may find ourselves separating from some of the sweetness of life for the sake of being "spiritual." Many people associate spirituality with being withdrawn and even a bit cranky. This, too, is a misconception. We are at once Divine *and* human; spirit dances together with nature, and its expression is joy!

With constant Remembrance of the Self, Vairagya, *all yearnings fade.*

What about those yearnings? Where do they all come from? How do they embed themselves so deeply in our thoughts and emotions? As newborns, we are in a constant state of *Vairagya,* easily remembering ourselves as Divine light. Our purity and innocence projects a wide-eyed, open-hearted sense of wonder. At the same time we experience an exquisite feeling of helplessness. Bathing, eating, dressing, moving our bodies, the most basic of care, is beyond our capacity. Yet we hold no judgments about the world, and neither accept nor reject the world's image of us. Slowly, we become more independent and are able to explore the world. We begin to understand criticism and find we are shrouded in judgments for such simple acts as soiling our diapers or dribbling when we eat our food. Our instruction book of do's and don'ts has begun to be written.

"Blue is for boys, pink is for girls."
"Girls play with dolls, boys play with trucks."
"People who come from this place are bad and steal."
"Only this school is good."

Confusion begins to occur at that young age, since we are still so closely identified with our Divine nature. Are we not in fact Divine Beings, and isn't everyone else also? Do I need to trade this Divine reality for earthly consciousness? Will this new set of rules eventually become my main reflection?

Our family and teachers continue to instill guidelines in us based on their own social understandings and prejudices. They feel it is their duty to do so, out of love for us and the desire to prepare us to live in society. Unfortunately, through the millennia, rules have taken precedence over love. As we internalize more traditions and social codes, we are forced into the lifelong balancing act of weighing our divinity against respect for society's rules.

THREE CHARACTERISTICS OF INDIVIDUAL CONSCIOUSNESS (CHITTA)

Through all these conditionings, the universal consciousness, or *chit,* remains the same. But as our material awareness flourishes, it begins to recede from us. The consciousness we retain is individual consciousness, or *chitta,* which is differentiated into three features: *buddhi, manas,* and *ahamkara.*

Buddhi functions as intellect and intuition, *manas* refers to sense perception, and *ahamkara* is the ego self-perceiving itself as a separate entity. Their cooperation allows us to reason, to perceive the world, to function, and to grow according to our individual needs.

The *buddhi,* as the discriminative and intuitive aspect, has no likes or dislikes. It stores information, and then relays it to the *manas* (senses) or to the *ahamkara* (ego-self). It harmoniously resonates with our inner knowing. The *buddhi* wants and needs nothing for itself, and is experienced as a clear reflection of consciousness. (The name Buddha, meaning "the enlightened one," is derived from the word *buddhi.*)

The *manas* functions as a receptor of sensual data. Our sight, hearing, taste, touch, and smell are governed by the *manas.* Unable to discriminate on its own, it feeds the sensory information back to the *buddhi* for clarification and validation, or to the *ahamkara* for action.

The *ahamkara* is the sense of "I, me, mine" that is commonly called the ego. This is the part that receives information from the *manas* (senses) and the *buddhi* (discrimination). It either desires or rejects their findings. "I want that" or "I don't want that." The ego has a poor reputation in spiritual circles as the part of our individual consciousness that divides and separates rather than unifies. In fact, we need a healthy ego to function in the physical world. When the ego is vibrant, it guides us to reflect our true nature, allowing the inner and outer worlds to flow together in harmony.

Perhaps, as you are walking down the street one fine day, you are feeling exceptionally content and in harmony with your surroundings. The *manas* begins to pick up a signal from the organ of sense—in this case, the nose—that a delicious smell is in the air. The smell begins to entice the sense of taste, causing your mouth to salivate. This alerts the *buddhi*, which then searches to identify the smell. "The odor is cinnamon, often used in cakes and pastries," the *buddhi* reports.

As your sensory involvement mounts, the eyes now engage with the words on a nearby window. The *buddhi* recognizes the word BAKERY. Now the vision, smell, and taste are involved in the discovery. The eyes spot a small, round spiral with little particles on top that appear sticky. The information is input and comes back identified as a "cinnamon bun with nuts."

Also stored in the *buddhi* is the resolve that you are not going to eat sugar for the next couple of weeks. Meanwhile the *ahamkara* (ego-self) has been enjoying the day and not paying much attention to what was going on, but with the perception of the sticky bun, it jumps into action. "Sticky bun?" The words suddenly summon its attention. "Where are there sticky buns?" Connecting immediately with the senses (*manas*) and ignoring the *buddhi* (discrimination), it informs the legs to march into the bakery. The hands seize a sticky bun and the *ahamkara* instructs the mouth to bite and chew it, finishing the tasty delight within seconds! Content once again, the *ahamkara* renews the resolve to "not eat sugar." This time it will have less power because it was so easily ignored. As we can see, all three aspects work together. The greatest influence will come from the one aspect of the three that has been strengthened and respected the most. If you allow discrimination and intuition to officiate, rather than trying only to satisfy your ego and senses, greater contentment will be the fruit.

But sometimes you may choose to override reason and follow your desires, as in the example above. Don't then feel guilty about your decision or agonize about how bad it is for you. This ruins the enjoyment of the moment and encourages negative effects on your health. Guilt *opposes* spiritual growth. If you make the decision to eat something you decided previously to avoid, then completely enjoy it! It is the ego that wanted it but now the ego is not letting you enjoy it! Instead, trick the ego and enjoy the experience.

Regret and guilt are just different forms of yearning—the yearning for the past, the yearning for another chance at a decision. Instead, remember yourself, and remember that you followed your own choice.

With constant Remembrance of the Self, Vairagya, *all yearnings fade*.

EXPERIENCING REMEMBERING THE SELF, *VAIRAGYA*

Make a list of what is important to you. People first, things next. Could the people and things on your list continue to be well cared for if you held the constant awareness that you are a Divine Being? By making this remembering a top priority, could you give even better care and love to others?

Maybe you and a friend are in a restaurant and you are insisting that she order your favorite dish. Consider how your mind and emotions would react as you are subsequently told that there is only one portion available. Your friend instantly says, "You have it; I can easily order something else." Do you insist that she has the dish or do you feel it is "yours"?

If that situation is too easy, try something more challenging. What type of reaction do you think you would have if you found out that someone less qualified than you received "your" promotion?

Or the person you really hoped would invite you to the biggest event of the year takes someone else?

Observe how you react to the many daily events in your own life.

As the remembrance that you are Divine takes deeper root in your consciousness, challenges may test your conviction.

Make sure to remember your True Self in all conditions!

1.16 *When consciousness unites, it remains clear and unaffected by the external changes of nature, the* gunas. *This is the ultimate* Vairagya.

The more we remember the Divine Self, the brighter the pure diamond light is reflected. Resting in that light, we are unaffected by external changes.

We again are called to look at the interplay of the three attributes of nature, or *gunas: Tamas* (inactivity), *Rajas* (overactivity), and *Sattwa* (balance), which we spoke about in Sutra I. 1. The world and everything in it constantly moves between these three states, but if we are able to remember the Self at all times, they are unable to influence us.

All nature, including us, reflects this continuous cyclic movement of time and change. The relentless play of the *gunas* is like waves crashing onto the shore and then rushing to merge back with the sea. It is often called the Sea of Samsara (the sea of birth and death). Helplessly caught in this illusion of tumultuous changes, we experience valuable lessons here on earth. As we long for steadiness and balance, we observe and then transcend the constant movement that inhibits us from reuniting with our essential nature.

OUR MINDS AND EMOTIONS COME IN TECHNICOLOR

When we identify with the *gunas* (rather than the True Self), the clear light within becomes prismatic, showering a rainbow of colors *(Varnas)* on the mind and emotions. This rainbow literally colors how we think and feel, and these colors are reflected in our common parlance. We might be feeling blue, seeing red, or turning green with envy.

Tamas, a state of inactivity, manifests itself most extremely as an inability to make decisions, or immobilizes us through fatigue or fear. A positive attribute of *Tamas* is its ability to draw us inward, allowing us to have deep, restful sleep at night.

Rajas, or overactivity, is a constant companion in our modern world, encouraging us to literally or figuratively run in a hundred different directions, and to experience as many of the infinite choices as possible. Primarily felt in the daytime hours, *Rajas* reaches its zenith at noon. All activity, including eating and digesting, is best accomplished when *Rajas* is supreme. The positive aspect of *Rajas* is that by trying many things and exploring many possibilities, the stasis of *Tamas* is sure to be defeated. The energy is now moving (if not in the most efficient way) and eventually a decision will be made, either by choice or through default.

Sattwa is when balance reigns. This could also be described as "dynamic stillness," a state in which motion and rest occur in perfect harmony.

During the interplay of *Tamas* and *Rajas,* one often becomes dominant while the other submits. Each comfortably rules its own domain.

Following the natural flow of the *gunas,* we live in balance. We are hindered when the *Rajas* and *Tamas* within us clash with the gentle flow of nature. Insomnia is a great example of this. The night, ruled by *Tamas,* is a time to go inward and rest. If at bedtime the mind is still racing in a *Rajasic* state, sleeplessness occurs. The busy mind, fed by *Rajas,* cannot surrender its activity to the needs of the body in *Tamas.* The body is then drawn into the *Rajasic* state as well, becoming restless and losing its much-needed time to cocoon. Allowing the mind to calm with quiet activities a few hours before bedtime, we more readily surrender to a great night's sleep, the ultimate *Tamas.*

When we overextend our energies during *Rajas* and fail to honor the indrawn time of night, *Tamas* will creep into our daylight hours. We may find ourselves tired or unable to think clearly, wanting to curl up and take a nap. Cloudy days that obscure the sun often invite *Tamas* to visit us.

At all times, to varying degrees, nature contains all three gunas. Ideally, we would like our temperament to settle into the quality of *Sattwa* all the time, but usually there is a great deal of fluctuation. There are times we may need to go well out of our way to invite *Sattwic* qualities back into our life. Once the invitation is accepted, the world becomes a harmonious venue for both action and inaction.

> "One is elevated in consciousness when one experiences
> action in inaction, and inaction in action."
>
> —*Bhagavad-Gita*

When consciousness unites, it remains clear and unaffected by the external changes of nature, the gunas. *This is the ultimate* Vairagya.

With continuous Yoga practice, the body, mind, and emotions are able to narrow the ranges of both *Tamas* and *Rajas.* With this limiting, *Sattwa* is revealed and the deeper practices begin to divulge their transformational effect.

THE MIND AND EMOTIONS AND THE MOON

To further help us understand this concept, imagine the moon and its cycles. From earth, the moon appears at certain times of the month to be half light and half dark. (It is actually difficult to see the half-dark portion, so it seems to be only half of the moon.) That is the time of *Sattwa,* a balance between dark and light. Within a few days the light increases until it fully illuminates the moon, and *Rajas* is present. With this full light of the moon, the mind and emotions are most active. Anyone who works at a hospital can attest to the chaos of a full moon. The patients are more restless and the emergency room is much fuller. Darkness then begins to obscure the light as the new moon, *Tamas,* begins to hold sway. With the dark or new moon, the mind and emotions are more indrawn; in extreme cases we may feel moody, or even depressed.

Tamas often masquerades as *Sattwa.* Did you ever mistake your lack of ambition, or even a bit of depression, for a feeling of stillness and contentment? Perhaps you were able to fool others, but deep inside you knew you couldn't be further from tranquillity. *Tamas* tends toward a lack of energetic consciousness, while *Sattwa* is an efficient and steady energy. When abiding in the *Tamasic guna,* we must transit through *Rajas* to embrace *Sattwa.*

If you're feeling lazy, a friend might encourage you to get up and *do something,* anything, to move the energy. Often hesitant to act because we are unwilling to make mistakes, we become immobilized *(Tamas).* By calling on *Rajas,* we may make many wrong turns, but at least we are moving. If after spinning our wheels we are able to spend a moment in stillness, we may discover that, miraculously, our center is rediscovered, and *Sattwa* is again with us.

With the glorious vision of the Self, nature's constantly changing temperament is unveiled. Through remembering, we honor the unchanging divinity in its eternal dance with our constantly changing humanity.

"If you become whole, everything will come to you."

—*Tao Te Ching*

When consciousness unites, it remains clear and unaffected by the external changes of nature, the gunas. *This is the ultimate* Vairagya.

EXPERIENCING THE EFFECT OF THE GUNAS (ATTRIBUTES OF NATURE) ON THE MIND AND EMOTIONS

Notice your mind and feelings throughout the day. Sometimes you may feel yourself turning inward, while at other times you are active and energetic.

Do you feel in harmony with the dominant guna *of the hour? Is that* guna *supporting you in what you need to do at that time?*

When you feel out of balance, identify which guna *you are in.*

Be still for a few minutes and imagine that you are coming into balance.

If you are feeling Tamasic, *do something active with your body, mind, or both.*

If you are a bit Rajasic, *do something to soothe yourself, like listening to quiet music or simply taking a few deep breaths.*

Resist the temptation to feed the guna *you are in. Ultimately, you will find a proven pathway to* Sattwa *as you discover ways to bring balance into your life.*

1.17 *By cultivation of Abhyasa and Vairagya, the intellect becomes keen, reasoning is clear, bliss is reflected to all, and outward identification unites with the Supreme Consciousness.*

1.18 *With continued awareness, we identify only with the pure consciousness residing in the heart.*

1.19 *Through identification with pure consciousness, the physical world can be transcended.*

1.20 *This identification is enhanced by faith, dynamism, intention, reflection, and perception.*

1.21 *To the dedicated and devoted, the Divine truth is revealed.*

1.22 *Spiritual Consciousness develops in direct proportion to one's dedication.*

BHAKTI YOGA:
Cultivating the Yoga of Devotion

*B*HAKTI YOGA, or the Yoga of Devotion, is one of the most accessible and enjoyable ways to merge with the infinite. For many of us this way of devotion is omnipresent and seamlessly meshes with our own temperament.

*Boundless love and devotion unite us with
the Divine Consciousness.*

The Divine Consciousness is self-effulgent like the sun.

The Divine is the essence of all knowledge, wisdom, and love.

*Knowledge, wisdom, and love are the omnipresent teachers,
in all beings.*

Repeating the sacred sound manifests Divine Consciousness.

*When expressed with great devotion, the sacred sound
reveals our Divine nature.*

By faithful repetition, the inner light luminously shines.

1.23 *Boundless love and devotion unite us with the Divine Consciousness.*

The secret to unleashing the power of devotion is now offered to us as *Bhakti Yoga.* Merging with the Divine through supreme devotion, *Iswara Pranidhana,* is such an important concept that we will see it repeated many more times in the *Yoga Sutras.*

THE EVER-BLOSSOMING WAY OF *BHAKTI*

Bhakti Yoga, often seen as a mysterious path of devotion, is offered by the *Yoga Sutras* in a systematic form. In fact, its message is simple, and it seems almost strange that something as natural as opening our hearts has to be taught. After all, we arrive in this world with an open heart. But if it is not nurtured, that openness diminishes and is often unable to live past the limited duration of childhood. The sutras encourage us to continually cultivate that precious gift.

Bhakti Yoga in its various forms is the most widely embraced practice in the world. Also *Bhakti,* not *Hatha,* is the most practiced form of Yoga! This may be because everyone, from the simple to the clever, can discover its secret to the heart.

Bhakti is often erroneously considered a path only for those possessing a highly emotional temperament. Images of weeping or chanting in rapture before an altar of the Divine are often associated with it. This is *one* aspect of *Bhakti* devotion, but be careful not to confuse *devotion* with *emotion.* True devotion and love shine through the Divine in every being.

Most of us traversing our particular way of devotion acknowledge that there is something beyond the individual "I." With an experience of great power, like standing on the shore of the boundless sea, or witnessing the birth of a baby, we are embraced by feelings of gratitude *and* humility. These experiences link us to our hearts.

Like tomorrow's beautiful flower encased in a delicate bud, the expanded heart is, for many of us, still in a latent form. The heart, like the bud, protects itself from the harshness of the external world by staying cocooned, locking the Divine within. But through the continuous nurturing of deep devotion, the bud, in guarded increments, can expand its petals to fully blossom in all its beauty.

"To love means never to be afraid of the windstorms of life;
should you shield the canyons from the windstorms you would
never see the beauty of the carvings."
—*Elisabeth Kübler-Ross*

*Boundless love and devotion unite us with the Divine
Consciousness.*

LEARNING TO LOVE LOVE

Unlike many of the practices that tend toward precise instructions, there is no right or wrong way to love. Each one of us, in our own way, can express our wholehearted love of the Divine and of creation. Often as we tread lightly on this glorious path, the heart embraces the Divine in external form. It is always interesting for me to speak to individuals of the same faith about their personal relationship with the Divine, and to notice how differently each experiences it—as mother, father, friend, or something else entirely. Some identify the Divine with a name and a form, yet for others it is nameless and formless. Many imagine cosmic consciousness somewhere far away in heaven; for others it takes on a more accessible human form.

Often the Divine speaks through a person or a holy book. Within the same holy book, the Divine is described as wrathful, and loving, and spiteful, and compassionate. Which one is accurate? Could it be that we are projecting our own human traits and personalities onto the Divine? Could the Divine embody all of these qualities? Choose carefully which aspect you want to embrace, for "As you think, so you become." Whatever way you decide to show your devotion, *Bhakti* is one of the most natural ways for us to locate the ever-present Divine.

From our outward devotion we discover that the Divine *also* dwells within. At first it may appear as a small part of us, usually through some altruistic act. On performing an act of kindness, we may give credit to that glimmer of the indwelling Divine. "It is not me," we say, gesturing toward the sky. What happens when we are blamed? Hanging our heads we refer to the dominant "human" perception of who we are and proclaim, "It's all my fault, I am not good enough."

Eventually, and perhaps after much discomfort, we arrive at the next stage of spiritual evolution, recognizing that, in good deeds and in bad, we are one with the Divine. The greatest challenge awaits us: to accept that the same Divine dwells in everyone!

A WOMAN'S HEART

Honored by most traditions, a compassionate heart has become the symbol for devotion. It is often a female heart that is used as the standard for that devotion and love. In even the youngest of girls, care and nurturing for even the smallest creatures are intuitive and natural.

Motherhood has been anointed the apex of this love and compassion. Madonna and child was a familiar theme in the Christian church, even during times when wrathful images of the Divine were common. Worshippers longed for a compassionate image to speak to their hearts, and to intercede with the angry father. In such times, the mother often soothes the child and the father as well. Cultivate loving devotion, and you may find that it transforms everyone around you.

A WOMAN'S TWO HEARTS

Women are graced with what is often referred to as the "womb heart." It relates to the "beating heart" through intuition and feelings. This legacy of love is so powerful that it is able to sustain a new life. The beating heart and womb heart each hold the sacred essence of consciousness. The capacity of our "beating" heart expands greatly as we experience infinite love; the overflow feeds us and others. To my joy, I found one ancient attempt in the Old Testament of the Bible to express the Divine as *Hiranya Garbha,* or the Golden Womb, the source of all beings that resides within each heart.

For many women, when the womb heart begins its metamorphosis to embrace a new life, the beating heart's capacity for love and devotion begins to expand. Our expectant mother now experiences three hearts within her: her beating heart, her womb heart, and the new soul's heart within her womb. Three pools of Divine love. Is it any wonder we feel radiance emanating from an expectant mother? Everyone is drawn to her, with all three of her hearts active; she is directly sourcing Divine love.

When it comes to love and devotion, motherhood holds the secret. Even those of us who have never physically given birth have within us the capacity and intuitive preparation for nurturing. All too often, in place of our heart's song, we listen to the intellectual values of our society cloaking our intuitive power. With grace, we can embrace both aspects, allowing the love and devotion to be channeled into the foundation of our lives.

Boundless love and devotion unite us with the Divine Consciousness.

One of the most sincere ways devotion can be expressed is through prayer. Try to find a time in your memory when you absent-mindedly repeated a prayer in your chosen place of worship. The words were being said, but they were probably being recited by the mouth, not the heart. For prayer to reach its full power, the heart must be the main speaker.

A HUMBLE OFFERING OF GREAT DEVOTION

In the twilight of the predawn hours, after taking a ritual bath, simple women in India gather cow patties. Chanting prayers, hearts overflowing with love and devotion, they roll the patties into sizable balls. After infusing the Divine into these animal waste products, they sweetly place a delicate flower on the crown of the mound. The women then make offerings of water, rice, and flower petals to further instill the Divine into the emerging form of Lord Ganesha, the elephant god and the remover of obstacles.

To those of us growing up in a Western society, this seems like a bizarre and unsanitary practice. If we look at it from this perspective, though, we miss the transformational aspect of simple devotion.

"Real Love is possible only when you see everything as yourself."
—*Sri Swami Satchidananda*

"When you drink the water, remember the spring from where it came."
—*Chinese proverb*

Boundless love and devotion unite us with the Divine Consciousness.

EXPERIENCING THE RHYTHM
OF YOUR TWO HEARTS

In a quiet room, sit or lie comfortably.

Choose a simple chant or prayer that touches your heart in a very deep way.

Place one hand on your beating heart and the other on your womb heart. (Even if your physical womb is not there, the energy can still be summoned.)

With deep breaths say the prayer aloud or silently, and begin to feel the energy in each of the two hearts.

Notice if the energy of each has a different quality.

As the breathing and chanting continue, can you feel a balance of energy between the two?

With the balance, experience the flow of love you feel for your own child or loved one.

Then slowly continue to expand that love to others as it eventually embraces all.

Stay resting in that balance for as long as you like.

You can come to this practice anytime during the day when you discover you are missing that feeling of love. This allows you to embrace the Divine in everyday life.

1.24 The Divine Consciousness is self-effulgent like the sun.

If the Divine is always in our hearts, then why would we need to do anything to call it forth? A contracted heart obscures the Divine within. With its opening, the Divine is revealed and we proclaim it as a miracle. The true miracle is that we are able to overcome doubt, and to experience that, with an open, loving heart, everything is possible.

The Divine Consciousness is self-effulgent like the sun.

1.25 The Divine is the essence of all knowledge, wisdom, and love.

1.26 Knowledge, wisdom, and love are the omnipresent teachers, in all beings.

In the ancient Yoga tradition, a spiritual teacher is called a *Sat Guru,* or teacher of truth. The word "guru" has two parts: "gu," that which hides our true light, and "ru," that which removes the covering. The word was traditionally reserved for a spiritual teacher of the highest regard; however, it has entered into common parlance, and can even be found in the business pages of a newspaper.

   Our mother is our first guru, teaching us the ways of love and of the world. Focused on her new treasure, she cares for us without judgment or expectations, and we are openly nourished by her infinite love. From the safety of our mother's heart, we are introduced to our father's wisdom. Later, our schoolteachers begin our study of the vast knowledge of the world. Eventually, the universe itself is revealed to us as our all-pervading teacher, a university of enormous proportions.

IS A TEACHER ALWAYS A GURU?

In our lifetime we encounter any number of "teachers" who guide and educate us. For this ordinary accumulation of knowledge, there are many well-trained *uppa gurus* (worldly teachers) available to us. Most of us have had the privilege of being taught by a few inspiring teachers, while other teachers made us bolt at the sound of the school bell's ring.

Worldly teachers learn their knowledge from books and from their own teachers. They pass this information forward, usually discouraged from adding their own flavor to the teachings. Prospective teachers are often taught not to interpret, just to stick to the facts as they learned them. Often the teacher is not an expert in the subject, but has a keen intellect that allows her or him to teach the subject so you can learn and refine your understanding.

These are fine attributes for an educator in the worldly sense, but not for a spiritual teacher. The spiritual guru must live what s/he teaches, as it is from truth that the power emanates.

Finding a true teacher in the uncharted territory of spirituality is challenging. Our relationship to the spiritual teacher requires enormous depth and commitment. We may be unable to grasp the vast scope of knowledge necessary to become awakened. Especially in these more skeptical times, the value of a living teacher is not appreciated. A true *Sat Guru* does not merely pass on her or his acquired knowledge; the guru also transmits *shakti* (energy) from her or his vast reserves, to help kindle our own spark.

My guru, Swami Satchidanandaji, would often describe himself as yogurt culture. We, the students, were the hot milk, warmed by the fire of our practices. At the prescribed time the guru would transmit some of his *shakti* energy to us by touching us on the top of the head, as if he were placing a little bit of live yogurt culture into milk. With that transmission of *shakti,* our own energy began to grow and our devotion nurtured it. The culture continued to mature, transforming the milk into yogurt, and moving our human consciousness closer to the Divine. In time, we are able to pass some of that culture to others. The guru initiates the student, who then becomes the guru and perpetuates the cycle. Yoga has for millennia been a tradition that directly transmits the power of its teachings from guru to disciple.

The Divine is the essence of all knowledge, wisdom, and love.

Knowledge, wisdom, and love are the omnipresent teachers, in all beings.

Choosing the right teacher is not always as easy as we would like. Place integrity at the top of the list when looking for a spiritual teacher. Many spiritual teachers reflect the teachings and their actions back to us through a mirror to show us who we truly are *and* the greatness that is our essential nature. Some show through their actions *exactly what you do not want to become.* Both are valuable. But much is also reported these days about gurus demanding that their students live an exemplary life, one that they themselves do not live. Before placing your total faith in a spiritual teacher, examine closely how s/he embodies the worldly *and* Divine traits you wish to emulate.

Another important aspect is to always seek out a teacher who wants you to outshine her or him, not one who hopes to keep you in the student role forever. Learn as much from the guru on as many levels of your being as you are able. Let her or him be the link that will take you back to the essence of all teachings: the light within your own heart. When that spark is ignited, a true *Sat Guru* will be clear in letting you know that is not her or his light that s/he has given to you; instead, s/he has assisted you in rediscovering the same light of the Divine that shines in all. The purpose of seeking and learning from a guru is not to be bound, but to be *free*.

"When the student is ready, the guru appears." This well-known saying is often followed by a worthwhile addition: "When the student is ready, the guru disappears!"

MAY THE GURU BE WITH YOU

It is not always necessary for the guru or teacher to be in physical proximity or even in the physical form to impart her or his *shakti*. Many evolved souls guide us from other physical locations and realms. The subtle knows no boundaries. Spiritual support can come from the next town or from the far-reaching vistas we are yet to explore. For example, Lord Jesus, Lord Buddha, Lord Siva, Sri Krishna, Sri Radha, Sri Durga, Sri Lakshmi, Kwan Yin, Mother Mary, and others have successfully inspired devotees to find their Divine essence for millennia. This is why the sutras say that the teacher of all teachers, the guru of gurus, is knowledge, wisdom, and love—boundless, eternal, pure, and unchanged by time.

> "Let your teacher be love itself."
>
> —*Rumi*

The Divine is the essence of all knowledge, wisdom, and love.

Knowledge, wisdom, and love are the omnipresent teachers, in all beings.

EXPERIENCING YOUR RELATIONSHIP TO THE
INTERNAL OR EXTERNAL GURU

Sit quietly and allow yourself to recall all the gurus and teachers who have taught you in the past and those who are guiding you now.

What lessons have you learned? How to act and how to be?

Were there some who showed you, by their words or actions, what not to do and how not to be?

Observing your present spiritual path, could a guru or a teacher enrich and increase the depth of your practice?

The first step in attracting a guru or a teacher is knowing that you are ready to receive guidance.

Set the intention and open your heart.

If you already have a guru or a teacher, are you able to accept the teachings wholeheartedly?

Does the guru or teacher live what s/he teaches?

Does s/he allow you to grow and flourish in your own personality?

Recommit yourself to knowledge, wisdom, and love as the ultimate teachers.

1.27 *Repeating the sacred sound manifests Divine Consciousness.*

We are very much a verbal society—the word, it is said, is "might-ier than the sword." The old adage "Sticks and stones will break my bones but words will never hurt me" is patently untrue today. Lawsuits for saying hurtful words about someone are rampant. We can feel the power of words in the way they affect our emotions. A kind one can leave a smile on our face for hours; a cruel one can bring us to tears. This power of words can be seen in Sacred Texts as well.

The *Rig Veda* tells us, "In the beginning was *Brahman* [Divine Consciousness] as the sound and this sound truly was the supreme *Brahman*." This is almost identical to the Bible: "In the beginning was the word, and the word was with God and the word *was* God."

Often, when we visit an ancient place of worship, we can feel a special vibration. Sitting in a temple or a church causes our minds and hearts to be uplifted. This is the effect of many thousands of devoted prayers that reverberate in sacred vibration through the atmosphere. Prayers in an ancient language radiate a special ele-vating quality when repeated with a focused mind and an open heart. Even if you visit a holy shrine that is not of your tradition, you will likely find a sublime comfort there.

From the beginning of time there have been vibrations, or pulsa-tions, which eventually formed audible sounds. The sacred sound vibration is called a mantra. A "*mantra*" is name *(nama),* form *(rupa),* and action (karma) of Divine Consciousness. These mantras often do not have a literal meaning, but in our need to engage the intellect, we may assign them "meanings." A mantra is intended to transcend the mind by invoking a celestial sound, transporting us to a higher level of understanding.

"Mantra" has found its way into common usage. It is used to mean a word that, when spoken, wields its own power and transcends thoughts, emotions, and our ordinary view of the world.

Repeating the sacred sound manifests Divine Consciousness.

REPEAT AS YOU LISTEN, LISTEN AS YOU REPEAT.

The ancient prayers and sacred sounds from each tradition are calls, encouraging us to embark on our journey to the Divine. "*Om*," "*Amen*," and "*Ameen*" all hold the heartfelt feeling of the Divine presence. Also, the peaceful vibrations of the Sanskrit "*Om Shanti*" mirror the Hebrew word for peace, "*Shalom*." These vibrations seem to unite us, even when our traditions diverge.

Love is a wonderful vibration to choose. How adored you feel when someone says the words "I love you!" Love resonates in all languages throughout the world. Say *love* in French, "*amour*," or Italian, "*amore*," or Spanish, "*amor*." Choose "love," or any phrase that, when repeated, reverberates within your entire being. Repeat it to yourself—one hundred, two hundred times a day.

This repetition of a sacred sound, word, or prayer is called *japa*. With each repetition, we become more in alignment with our true nature. When we hear it, see it, and say it, our bodies, minds, and worlds expand as the inner light is sparked.

"OM": THE SACRED SOUND OF UNIVERSAL CONSCIOUSNESS

"*Om*" is the sacred mantra of divinity. It is chanted and revered as the sound from which all other sounds resonate, awakening universal consciousness. In this way it is the guru of sounds, invoking the Divine Consciousness in every sound.

The *Mandukaya Upanishad* expounds on the meaning of *"Om,"* attempting to explain the simple essence of that sound. It divides *"Om"* into four sounds and stages. *A, U, M,* and the sound that is beyond all verbal pronunciation.

A is the beginning of all sounds. This is usually a baby's first sound, made simply by opening the mouth and saying "Ah." The sound comes from the back of the tongue. Next the *U* sound, like *OO,* is formed, moving forward in the mouth. And then, with the lips and teeth closed, the *M* is hummed.

A-U-M forms a trinity similar to other trinities that are more familiar: body-mind-spirit, creator-preserver-destroyer, past-present-future, the three *gunas,* or Mother, Father, God, the Holy Trinity, and on and on. It brings all three prongs together in a simple sound.

Going beyond the trinity, the last bit of breath after the *"Om"* continues to be released without an audible sound to accompany it. This fourth part of *"Om"* is the unspoken sound, *anahatha.* It is the vibration before and after all sound. If we listen closely after chanting, the resonance of the *mmm* sound can be felt, sometimes constant and sometimes oscillating. It is the sound of our merging with the infinite. This is the *Pranava,* the sound of *Prana,* the Divine energy.

All other *Sanskrit* mantras radiate from the root vibration *"Om."* Since *"Om"* is so subtle, other mantric vibrations are often added to allow the mantra to be more easily experienced. *"Om Shanti"* and *"Om Namah Sivaya"* are examples of this.

After a time of constant repetition, *japa,* the mantra will begin to repeat seemingly by itself. At that time we enjoy listening. This listening is called *ajapa.* It is the sound of universal power rejuvenating itself.

With *japa,* the cells in our body and mind vibrate with that chosen sound as we assume the qualities. Today we have graphic machines that draw geometric patterns when certain sounds are produced. This concept existed centuries before in the yogic practice of repeating a mantra. When the sound *"Om"* and related mantras are chanted, a pattern is formed called a yantra (or often called mandala). Yogis saw and then reproduced these sacred drawings on paper and stone from their third eye. Even today the use of yantras as aids for focusing and meditation is honored.

> "Truth is one, many are the paths."
>
> —*Vedas*

Repeating the sacred sound manifests Divine Consciousness.

EXPERIENCING *"OM"* AS DIVINE CONSCIOUSNESS BY REPEATING AND LISTENING

Sit quietly and comfortably either on a chair or on the floor.

Align your head, neck, and spine. Expand your heart center.

Take in a few deep breaths to calm the body, mind, and emotions.

Begin to chant the sacred mantra "Om" four distinct ways.

First, inhale deeply and pronounce the O longer than the M: OOOOOOOMMM.

This enlivens the earth chakras (energy centers) and allows us a feeling of groundedness.

Repeat several times.

Second, inhale deeply and give the O and M sounds equal length: OOOOOMMMMM.

This brings balance to the earth and higher chakras.

Repeat several times.

Third, inhale deeply and elongate the M sound: OOOMMMM.

This brings awareness to the higher chakras for meditation.

Repeat several times.

Fourth, inhale deeply and chant "OM" with the elongated M as before. Then allow the breath to complete its exhalation without any audible sound, only listening: OOOMMMMM . . . .

This allows awareness to move to the highest levels of consciousness.

Repeat several times.

Be still and listen, and know that you are Divine.

1.28 *When expressed with great devotion, the sacred sound reveals our Divine nature.*

The sacred sound must pluck the strings of our heart in order to unite our entire being. Often we are accustomed to repeating the same prayer, with our mind and heart engaged elsewhere. Then the prayer is only given lip service. The real grace comes when we are unified on all levels of our being.

When expressed with great devotion, the sacred sound reveals our Divine nature.

1.29 *By faithful repetition, the inner light luminously shines.*

The real secret is to have a full and open heart when repeating a mantra or engaging in any spiritual practice. In the beginning, we are very concerned about correctly pronouncing the mantra or prayer. We may be "doing it exactly right," yet it may lack the most essential ingredient, devotion. The real power comes from the heart.

By faithful repetition, the inner light luminously shines.

EXPERIENCING YOUR HEART'S SONG

Sit comfortably in a chair or on the floor.

Choose a mantra or a prayer that allows your heart to fill with love. It does not matter if you do not know the meaning. The feeling is most important.

Begin to repeat this sacred sound aloud in a soft voice.

When, after some time, you are accustomed to the sound and feeling of the vibration, permit the lips and tongue to repeat the word delicately and thoughtfully, in a heartfelt whisper.

Moving further in, allow the heart to repeat it in silence. Feel the vibration moving in and out of your heart with each pulsation. Continue for a few minutes.

*Allow the heart to overflow with the vibration and nourish your
entire being. As you continue your day, the mantra will continue
to repeat with each beat of your heart.*

*Feel that it is near and dear to you. Be faithful to it, and it will
give you the secret to the power of the universe.*

THE FOUR LOCKS AND FOUR KEYS:
Sustaining Equanimity

These sutras speak about the potential imbalances we may encounter on the physical, mental, and emotional levels. They obscure the knowledge of our true nature. Offered are various ways to prevent these imbalances as well as ways to regain that precarious balance, if lost.

They show why the spiritual path is often likened to walking on a razor's edge.

Perception of our true nature is often obscured by physical, mental, and emotional imbalances.

These imbalances can promote restlessness, uneven breathing, worry, and loss of hope.

These imbalances can be prevented from engaging by developing loyalty to a sacred practice.

To preserve openness of heart and calmness of mind, nurture these attitudes:

Kindness to those who are happy
Compassion for those who are less fortunate
Honor for those who embody noble qualities
Equanimity to those whose actions oppose your values.

Slow, easeful exhalations can be used to restore
and preserve balance.

Or engage the focus on an inspiring object.

Or cultivate devotion to the supreme, ever-blissful Light within.

Or receive grace from a great soul, who exudes Divine qualities.

Or reflect on a peaceful feeling from an experience,
a dream, or deep sleep.

Or dedicate yourself to anything that elevates
and embraces your heart.

1.30 *Perception of our true nature is often obscured by physical, mental, and emotional imbalances.*

1.31 *These imbalances can promote restlessness, uneven breathing, worry, and loss of hope.*

1.32 *These imbalances can be prevented from engaging by developing loyalty to a sacred practice.*

These sutras are understandable and do not seem to need further commentary. (They may be not as easy to put into practice as they are to comprehend!)

1.33 *To preserve openness of heart and calmness of mind, nurture these attitudes:*

Kindness to those who are happy
Compassion for those who are less fortunate
Honor for those who embody noble qualities
Equanimity to those whose actions oppose your values.

This is a large dose of practical advice that allows us to integrate the highest spiritual values into our everyday lives. When we engage in the more "formal practices," that is, postures, breathing, or sitting in meditation, distractions often occur. We are affected by these distractions; however, they are more manageable when confined to our private world. Once we leave our sanctified space, the intrusions of the larger world present us with many more challenges.

Here we are offered four priceless keys that if used in conjunction with the correct locks open portals that enable us to retain our inner peace in all circumstances. The greatest challenge is to remember that *we hold the keys to our own peace*.

At first reading this sutra, we may think, "This is easy—of course I would react that way." As we begin to apply these subtle principles to our daily lives, we can trick ourselves into believing that we are kinder and more compassionate than we actually are. The ease manifests when thought, word, *and* deed mesh together.

These keys are also useful when reacting to our own actions, which can be even more complex than other people's actions. As the judging mind barges in, can the heart supersede it? Let's look at what a few of the challenges might be like. Of course, allow these to serve as examples that can help you explore the challenges in your own life.

Kindness to those who are happy.

Imagine that you are meeting a friend whom you have not seen in ages. You pack a picnic and head to the park to catch up on what is happening in her life. Finding an ideal spot, you spread out a blanket, lay out the food, and begin to enjoy the tasty dishes and the wonderful company.

After the first two bites, both body and heart feel nourished. Just then a man sits down very close to you and lights up a big, fat, juicy cigar. Puffing happily, he leans back in the grass with a big grin, allowing the billowing smoke to waft directly into your nose and onto your food.

Before taking any action, observe your mind. Are you annoyed, even angry? "Who is *he* to ruin my perfect time by polluting us with cigar toxin!" Is judgment creeping in? Are you thinking how unconscious he must be to do something like that! "Is he doing it purposely to annoy me?"

Your blood pressure has probably risen, and your immune function is already weakened—not from the cigar toxin, but from your own emotions and thoughts that have taken control.

Now, give the heart a chance and look again at the man and the situation. He seems happy, relaxed, and at ease with the world, enjoying his treat. Do you want to spoil the mood and your own special time by responding to the situation with anger and self-righteousness? Those two emotions in particular can take hours to recover from.

Instead, try opening your heart and allowing kindness to meet his happiness. With a kind vibration, let the man know that you are happy he is enjoying his expensive cigar. Since you also would like to enjoy your meal, would he mind directing the smoke in another direction, or even better, enjoying it in another location? His response will often match the energy as well as the words you put forth.

Most situations in your life are not as dramatic, yet the same remedy will apply. Try overriding the mind's indignation with the heart's desire to love everyone. You may be amazed at the results.

Compassion for those who are less fortunate.

The word "compassion" is such a beautiful word; soft and gentle, it is comprised of two parts: *com*, meaning "with," and *passion*, meaning "any intense emotion, either pleasurable or painful." Many times it is difficult to know which aspect of passion we are feeling, and sometimes we clearly encounter both at the same time.

Compassion is a form of infinite love, in that nothing can affect or limit it. It is extolled as a virtue for the very few, but is it? As women we seem to have a natural gift for radiating love and compassion. Our heartfelt compassion often embraces people in unfortunate circumstances beyond their control.

What, then, could prevail that would obscure this natural quality? In certain circumstances a hesitation on our part may occur when someone is unhappy and needs our compassionate balm. Could our own worry and stress place compassion on the back burner?

Running late might be reason enough to create anxiety and prompt us to neglect our compassionate nature. If you feel rushed, a simple delay accelerates your anxiety. I think everyone has had this experience: you're waiting at a red light. Right as it changes to green, your foot comes off the brake, hovering above the gas pedal— you're ready to go! But traffic is not moving! Irritation mounts. You strain to look out the window, even give a toot on the horn. "Why are they not moving? The light is not going to get any greener! Probably someone's daydreaming, or talking on her cell phone. I don't have all day! Let's go!!" You're now in a fully adrenaline-charged state.

Imagine that when accelerating forcefully as the light turns from yellow to red, you notice out of the corner of your eye a blind woman and her guide dog safely finishing traversing the street. *That was the cause of the delay*—the very delay that caused you to be so irritated, anxious, and even angry. Observing the woman and her dog, your heart is again able to open and expand. The anger and annoyance dissipate, replaced by compassion.

The next time, in a similar situation, recall this story and give the benefit of the doubt, allowing compassion to take over the driver's seat.

Compassion for those who are less fortunate.

Once we decide a person has a genuine reason for her suffering, our scope of compassion waxes and wanes according to how much we feel she "caused her own problem." Let's say that after getting fired from her third job, your friend comes to you for a compassionate ear. Each time she was fired, it was because she "borrowed" money from petty cash and was discovered. Your mind is thinking, "Well, she did it, *and* she got caught! She's smarter than that; why would she do such a thing? She doesn't need the money that much, does she?" Running wild with judgment and castigation, you plan your speech, based on "tough love." But she has already been reprimanded and suffered humiliation due to her actions. Out of work and defeated, she came to you seeking compassion and love. This is a perfect time to step back from the situation and reevaluate your role. Let your heart softly interrupt the blaming process and observe, "She seems so unhappy. Her heart is sad. She feels rejected and embarrassed, and knows the next job will be harder to land because of her now very blemished record." Your part is to soothe her with a compassionate balm, rather than play a parental role and teach her a lesson. Whatever action people take, whether you approve of it or not, always make sure they know that you love them.

"Through compassion you find that all human beings are just like you."
—His Holiness the Dalai Lama

Compassion for those who are less fortunate.

The way we treat others often reflects on how we treat ourselves. When we are compassionate to those around us, it becomes easier to replicate that compassion when we are the one who caused a problem.

Did you ever press the wrong button on the computer and delete hours of work? Or perhaps you thought you set the oven to go on at a certain time but your dinner guests arrived to find dinner uncooked? At times like this, and in even more serious situations, having compassion for yourself is most important. Instead of calling yourself unkind names, take a moment to speak sweetly, as if to a child. "It's okay, sweetie, we can always call for takeout." This is when you need all the love and compassion you can soak up. For many of us, compassion is a one-way street going out of ourselves. Let it circle back around; use compassion as a soothing salve to treat everyone, starting with yourself!

> "Compassion for myself is the most powerful healer of them all."
> —*Theodore Isaac Rubin*

Honor for those who embody noble qualities.

Thanks to electronic news media, magazines, books, and the Internet, historical information is in abundance, and most of us are fortunate to learn of great souls and their accomplishments. The opportunity for inspiration seems boundless. As we rejoice in and appreciate their qualities, we are inspired by knowing that such greatness is possible. If this dynamic feat can be done by one, why not by others? Much of what we need to achieve the extraordinary is encouragement and inspiration. The rest seems to take care of itself.

Who are some of these great souls? We can probably agree on quite a few. Mother Teresa, Martin Luther King Jr., Mahatma Gandhi, Nelson Mandela, and others inspired miracles in our world. Through them and their deeds, the whole of humanity is elevated. There are also countless uncelebrated heroines and heroes among us, living their virtue quietly, who we know little about.

Everyone has human limitations along with her or his greatness; it is up to us to choose which aspects to focus on. Observing noble qualities in others is a virtue of the heart. Our own horizons expand as we look toward the highest in others. Feeling discouraged, we may deflate our own talents while putting others on pedestals. "Oh, she is so talented; I could never dance like that." "She is such a good cook. I always burn anything I bake." Or in our insecurity we find reason to bring them down beneath us. "Yes, she might be an extraordinary leader, but she is so wrapped up in her work that she neglects her family."

Instead, try to find noble qualities in everyone. Some of us may need to become archaeologists and dig deep. It could be as simple as the graceful way she picks up a flower, or her keen fashion sense, or his good work ethic. Whatever it is, no matter how simple it may seem, focusing on this virtue will create a pathway to our heart. The more we practice this way of relating to others, the easier it is to recognize their Divine qualities and ultimately ours, too.

Spiritual teachers are everywhere, if our hearts are conditioned to recognize them. These "ordinary people" have allowed me some of my most precious learning experiences.

Equanimity to those whose actions oppose your values.

There are people and situations that make our blood pressure spike by the mere mention of them. Certainly when we are offended by cruel or brutal acts, we feel we have the right to judge and then seek retribution.

It would be a wonderful world if all people acted with honor and consciousness. That, unfortunately, does not seem to be the way of life in this age. We ourselves, at times, may have acted, spoken, or thought unkindly, or hurt another person. Yet, we are eager to condemn, judge, and criticize others for doing so.

The Divine is present even in those who do unmentionable atrocities. Granted, it is sometimes very hard to locate the Divine in such people. Their minds and emotions are so disturbed and clouded, it is difficult to perceive the goodness that resides within them. For retaining *our* openness of heart and calmness of mind, we must learn to forgive even the unforgivable.

> "The ultimate measure of a person is not where they stand
> in moments of comfort and convenience, but where they stand
> in times of challenge and controversy."
> —*Dr. Martin Luther King Jr.*

The virtue of forgiveness is often misunderstood. There is a reluctance to grant it, for fear that it will let the offender "off the hook." But in truth, forgiveness is a natural stepping-stone to compassion. It gives us the opportunity to free others and ourselves. To hold hatred in our hearts is to clamp them tightly closed. Though the wrongdoer may feel the effects of our hate, we often suffer the most if we encase it within our hearts for too long. It erodes the very fiber of our love. It also binds us to the person we are condemning. By dwelling on the situation, we continually affirm that those who wronged us actually had the power to hurt us. This allows them to continue to hurt us! They become the object of our unkind focus. It is for our benefit, more so than for theirs, to see them as Divine Beings.

Forgiveness is a soothing balm vital to our health and happiness. If we grudgingly forgive, we still deem the other person responsible. "They did this to me, *but* I (in my generosity) will forgive them." As the heart softens through forgiveness, the understanding emerges that they are also hurt and unhappy, and then forgiveness melts into compassion.

Through compassion the identification of someone else as the perpetrator of our hurt vanishes. We understand that it is our perception that harms or heals. The same benevolent light shines within that person's heart as shines within ours.

To preserve openness of heart and calmness of mind, nurture these attitudes:

Kindness to those who are happy
Compassion for those who are less fortunate
Honor for those who embody noble qualities
Equanimity to those whose actions oppose your values.

EXPERIENCING USING THE RIGHT KEY
TO UNLOCK THE ATTITUDE TO PRESERVE
OPENNESS OF HEART AND CALMNESS OF MIND

At the end of each day, take a few minutes to review the attitudes that you used freely.

Was there a situation where you applied the incorrect "key" and it did not unlock a feeling of peace?

Yet, perhaps in another situation, the correct key opened to an unexpected feeling of calmness.

In a journal write down the lessons as you experienced them.

Reinforce the attitudes that you would like to incorporate into your life and alter the ones that no longer fit who you want to be.

Continue for several weeks and then appreciate how you have blossomed.

1.34 *Slow, easeful exhalations can be used to restore and preserve balance.*

1.35 *Or engage the focus on an inspiring object.*

1.36 *Or cultivate devotion to the supreme, ever-blissful Light within.*

1.37 *Or receive grace from a great soul, who exudes Divine qualities.*

1.38 *Or reflect on a peaceful feeling from an experience, a dream, or deep sleep.*

Retaining our balance and restoring it if lost are of utmost importance to our spiritual life. Recognizing that imbalance is the first step. Fortunately, once we know we are tipping that delicate balance, there are many ways to help restore our equilibrium. These sutras speak for themselves, giving us the guidance to regain our balance.

1.39 *Or dedicate yourself to anything that elevates and embraces your heart.*

Here we are given carte blanche to choose anything to which we want to dedicate our hearts. The preceding sutras have generously given us many wonderful suggestions for focusing the mind and the heart. Most people will find a suitable choice from within that group. If you do not find one that unlocks *your* heart, the sutras now invite you to create your own using two guiding principles.

First, choose something that will elevate you just by invoking its presence. And second, choose something that you love dearly and embrace it fully in your heart. If you are sincere and dedicated, you will be transported to its Divine qualities and from there your inner peace will be unveiled. These are sure recipes for success in spiritual practice.

Or dedicate yourself to anything that elevates and embraces your heart.

SAMADHI:
Merging with the
Divine Consciousness

FROM this sutra to the end of Book I, we are introduced to the grand rewards of having focused our awareness on the highest, which then merges into varying states of union with our Divine Consciousness (*Samadhi*). The stages of *Samadhi* reflect the progressive withdrawal of individual consciousness (*chitta*) into the ocean of Universal Consciousness (*chit*). The various stages of the journey are presented in these sutras. (We will revisit *Samadhi* in Book III, Sutra 3.)

Gradually through focused awareness one's knowledge extends from the smallest atom to the greatest magnitude.

As a naturally pure crystal appears to take the color of everything around it yet remains unchanged, the yogi's heart remains pure and unaffected by its surroundings while attaining a state of oneness with all. This is Samadhi.

When awareness merges with a "material" object or form, if the name, quality, *and* knowledge *are perceived, this is* Savitarka Samadhi, *or reflective* Samadhi.

When awareness merges with a "material" object or form,
if knowledge alone *is perceived, this is* Nirvitarka Samadhi,
or spontaneous Samadhi.

When awareness merges with a "subtle" object or form,
two different Samadhis *are present,* Savichara *(perceiving*
name, quality, *and* knowledge*) and* Nirvichara *(perceiving*
knowledge alone*).*

These states of Samadhi *have the power to extend beyond all*
the "material" and "subtle" forms and objects, to reveal nature
in her unmanifested form.

All the Samadhis *described thus far have been* Sabija
(with seed), which have the ability to germinate, returning
us to ordinary consciousness.

In the purity of Nirvichara Samadhi, *Divine Consciousness*
becomes luminescent.

When consciousness dwells in absolute true knowledge
(Ritambhara Prajna), *direct spiritual perception dawns.*

This absolute true knowledge (Ritambhara Prajna)
is totally different from the knowledge gained by personal
experience, inference, and insights from the wise.

When experiencing this absolute true knowledge
(Ritambhara Prajna), *all previous* Samskaras *(impressions)*
are left behind and new ones are prevented from sprouting.

Nirbija *(seedless)* Samadhi *outshines all impressions*
and manifestations.

1.40 *Gradually through focused awareness one's knowledge extends from the smallest atom to the greatest magnitude.*

Here we are inspired by the benefits that come from our diligent spiritual practice. Up to now the focused mind and emotions were directed toward an object or form. These practices allowed us to attain the spiritual power necessary for the next stage of elevating consciousness, *Samadhi*.

The hidden secrets of the universe may now be revealed to us. They could be the essence of the smallest atom or the most distant star. This does not occur through observation or theory. Rather, when we know ourselves, all other forms and objects are known to us. We understand that we are all one.

> "By knowing the one, we know everything."
>
> —*Vedas*

Gradually through focused awareness one's knowledge extends from the smallest atom to the greatest magnitude.

1.41 *As a naturally pure crystal appears to take the color of everything around it yet remains unchanged, the yogi's heart remains pure and unaffected by its surroundings while attaining a state of oneness with all. This is* Samadhi.

This realization is the fulfillment of the concept of *Vairagya* (Remembrance of the Self) described in Book I, Sutra 15. When we hold fast to remembering we are the Divine Self, we merge with that Self. Even if the mind and emotions are temporarily distracted, the truth draws us back to the Self.

This sutra compares our consciousness to a perfectly clear crystal. When placed on a red cloth, it appears to be red. Once it is removed from the cloth, the flawless crystal is completely colorless again. We can repeat the action with a cloth of any color. Each time we can see that the color, which seemed to affect the crystal, in fact remains with the cloth. The crystal continues to reflect its true nature of purity and clarity.

Similarly, when we embrace the glory of knowing the Divine Self, our hearts and minds may appear to take on other characteristics. Yet, as soon as we remember our True Self, there is immediate and complete recognition of the pure and unchanging Divine.

A great and mighty queen once gave an audience to a man whose immediate response was to ridicule the queen's way of governing the country. After a polite amount of time, she began to speak, interrupting his ranting.

"How would *you* react," she said with kindness, "if you brought me an enormous basket of the finest fruits and I said, 'No, thank you, I am not interested in keeping your gift.'" A bit startled, the man stammered, "It would distress me to think that you did not like my gift, but I would take back the basket of fruits and leave."

"Very well," said the queen, calmly. "You have brought me a large basket of insults. Please take them away, as I do not wish to accept your offering."

In this story the queen took refuge in her true essence, remaining tranquil and secure even while the insults were attempting to cover her like a cloth. Each of us, like the queen, encounters people and things that try to coax us from the truth of knowing who we are. When we embrace this ever-present truth, we are free to live in joy within a constantly changing reality.

As a naturally pure crystal appears to take the color of everything around it yet remains unchanged, the yogi's heart remains pure and unaffected by its surroundings while attaining a state of oneness with all. This is Samadhi.

EXPERIENCING THE HEART AS A PURE CRYSTAL

Sit quietly and, with focused awareness, imagine your heart as a pure crystal.

Appreciate its clear, reflective quality.

Now begin to remember a situation or emotion. If possible, place a color value on it. (If it made you angry, for instance, it might reflect red.)

Slowly bring the situation or emotion, reflected in the color, near the pure crystal of your heart.

Notice if the crystal is affected by the color. Is the heart affected by the situation? Do your feelings release a color?

Observe if the mind and emotions engage and support the situation or the clarity of the heart crystal.

Now with great care remove the situation and the color from the crystal's reflection.

Does the heart crystal hold any of the color or has it stayed true to its pure and reflective nature?

Use this frequently to remember your true Divine Nature.

1.42 *When awareness merges with a "material" object or form, if the* name, quality, *and* knowledge *are perceived, this is* Savitarka Samadhi, *or reflective* Samadhi.

Once we have ascended through *Dharana,* contemplation, and *Dhyana,* meditation (Book III, Sutras 1–2), our awareness, inspired by the various suggestions offered in the previous sutras, is able to merge with the "material" object or form we have chosen. This is *Savitarka,* the first stage of *Samadhi.*

In *Savitarka Samadhi,* the awareness no longer wanders from the object itself (as it did in *Dharana* and *Dhyana*); instead it flutters between the name of the object, its quality, and the knowledge enveloped in the object.

In its simplest form, if we join our focused awareness to a candle flame ("material" object), we have identified it by its *name,* flame. We recognize the *qualities* of light and heat. The *knowledge* of the flame relates to our own observation that it gives light. After identifying all three attributes, our thoughts and feelings begin to wander, in an inconsistent pattern, to *name, quality,* and the *knowledge* it holds. With each new visit to one aspect or another, new variations will emerge. This keeps the mind and emotions engaged in movement.

Because the movements are slight, our focus is able to deepen and we alight in *Savitarka Samadhi.* Reaching this stage is a grace, which is enhanced by a feeling of gratitude. The constant wavering, although negligible, is enough to prevent us from attaining the state of full transcendental awareness.

When awareness merges with a "material" object or form, if the name, quality, *and* knowledge *are perceived, this is* Savitarka Samadhi, *or reflective* Samadhi.

1.43 *When awareness merges with a "material" object or form, if* knowledge alone *is perceived, this is* Nirvitarka Samadhi, *or spontaneous* Samadhi.

In this stage of *Samadhi,* identification with the "material" form of an object (its name and quality) retreats, and knowledge is all that remains. The awareness no longer wanders but merges with the essential perception of the "material" form or object.

Using the example of the candle flame, the identification with the name "flame" or even the quality of "light or heat" is absent in *Nirvitarka Samadhi.* Instead a higher knowledge beyond the senses allows us to know its unseen characteristics. We have acquired knowledge of the origin and purpose of its light.

Albert Einstein, the great scientist and visionary, was often asked how he discovered the intimate properties of something as subtle as light. His humble reply continues to inspire many. "I did not discover it, I meditated on it, until it revealed itself to me." It was not the laboratory testing that led to the discovery as much as the many years spent contemplating and meditating on the secrets concealed in light. When he ultimately merged with light in *Nirvitarka Samadhi,* all its secrets were revealed.

With *Nirvitarka Samadhi* we boldly enter the realm of mystical understanding, encountering a web of intricacies that are beyond the grasp of the logical mind.

When awareness merges with a "material" object or form, if knowledge alone *is perceived, this is* Nirvitarka Samadhi, *or spontaneous* Samadhi.

EXPERIENCING MERGING AWARENESS WITH A "MATERIAL" OBJECT OR FORM

(Please note: This practice is presented to help us to understand *Savitarka* and *Nirvitarka Samadhi*. It is not intended to induce the state itself. If it does occur, however, it is known as *grace*.)

Sit comfortably with a lit candle at eye level.

Begin to repeat the name "flame" in silent repetition.

Feel the quality of heat and light that the flame emits.

Experience the secret knowledge of how light emanates from the flame.

Then go back over the three parts, allowing the thoughts and feelings to stay with three attributes.

Notice when the awareness wanders, and gently refocus on the name, quality, and knowledge of the flame.

Let the name and quality fade and perceive only the essence of clear light.

As you return to material awareness, notice where your consciousness has led you.

1.44 *When awareness merges with a "subtle" object or form, two different* Samadhis *are present,* Savichara (*perceiving* name, quality, *and* knowledge) *and* Nirvichara (*perceiving* knowledge alone).

These are both higher stages of *Samadhi* than those previously discussed. With both *Savitarka* and *Nirvitarka Samadhi,* we are obliged by language and our five senses to present the concept of a "material" object or form in order to access its knowledge.

With both *Savichara* and *Nirvichara Samadhi,* knowledge is gained through merging awareness with "subtle" forms and objects. In *Savichara Samadhi,* there is again a vacillation between *name, quality,* and *knowledge;* the three remain separate, without blending. In *Nirvichara Samadhi, name* and *quality* blend, releasing *knowledge* alone to merge with our awareness.

These *Samadhis* are more difficult to comprehend as they are out of the ordinary confines of language and out of time and space as we know it. Being subtler, they elicit a deeper focus to reveal their essence.

Some examples include meditating on: a sacred mantra (especially in the ancient Sanskrit language); the chakras (energy vortexes), which hold thought, emotional patterns, and karmic forecasts; or one of the five subtle elements (*Tanmatras*) housed in the chakras. These "subtle" forms and objects may also include elevated thought or emotional forms, such as love, compassion, intuition, and so on.

For an example, the *Anahatha* chakra (heart chakra) is in the "subtle" rather than the "material" form and cannot be experienced through our five external senses. We are, however, able to merge awareness with the *Anahatha* chakra as a vessel emanating infinite love and compassion and experience that love and compassion in our lives. This is *Savichara Samadhi.*

When infinite love and compassion are experienced and nothing else fills the awareness, *Nirvichara Samadhi* is experienced.

This new level of consciousness is without cause or effect, place or time. The inexpressible states of pure bliss (*Sa-ananda Samadhi*) and the effulgence of the pure self (*Sa-asmita Samadhi*) that follow *Nirvichara Samadhi* allow us to radiate infinite love and compassion to all.

When awareness merges with a "subtle" object or form, two different Samadhis *are present*, Savichara (*perceiving* name, quality, *and* knowledge) *and* Nirvichara (*perceiving* knowledge alone).

EXPERIENCING MERGING AWARENESS WITH A "SUBTLE" OBJECT OR FORM

(Please note: This practice is to help us to understand *Savichara* and *Nirvichara Samadhi*. It is not intended to induce the state itself. If it does occur, however, it is known as *grace*.)

Sit comfortably.

Begin to repeat the name "Anahatha *chakra" silently.*

Feel the quality of infinite love and compassion this chakra emanates from the center of your heart.

Allow the knowledge of how love and compassion emanate from the Anahatha *chakra to come to you.*

Allow the thoughts and feelings to merge awareness with the name, quality, and knowledge of the Anahatha *chakra.*

Let the name and quality fade and allow yourself to be bathed in the knowledge of infinite love and compassion, the essence of the Anahatha chakra.

As you return to material awareness, notice where your consciousness has led you.

1.45 *These states of* Samadhi *have the power to extend beyond all the "material" and "subtle" forms and objects, to reveal nature in her unmanifested form.*

Our awareness becomes focused first on the "material" and then on the "subtle" elements. Their far-reaching power leads us to the essence of manifested energy and then to nature in her unmanifested form *(prakriti).* Here is where we meet the three *gunas* (attributes of nature) equal and in balance with one another.

With the slightest fluctuation, the delicate balance of energy is reordered, resulting in the manifestation of all-phenomenal matter (creation). So even in these elevated stages of *Samadhi,* we are still unable to merge completely with the True Self. In order for us to directly unite with the Divine, we must traverse and then transcend the phenomenal worlds, both manifested and unmanifested.

These states of Samadhi *have the power to extend beyond all the "material" and "subtle" forms and objects, to reveal nature in her unmanifested form.*

1.46 *All the* Samadhis *described thus far have been*
Sabija *(with seed), which have the ability to germinate,*
returning us to ordinary consciousness.

We have climbed the lofty stages of *Samadhi* only to learn of its
impermanence. The term *Sabija* (with seed) reminds us that the
bliss of this higher state is temporary, and our ordinary ways of
thinking and feeling can reappear at any moment.

Although these *Samadhis* are of a higher order than most of our
spiritual practices, they still have only a limited amount of power to
sustain consciousness in that exalted state for an extended time.
It can last for minutes or days, but at some point our awareness
returns to individual consciousness. This is due to the fertile seeds
holding our thoughts, emotions, and karmas. (Karma will be
described in Book II, Sutras 12–14.) However, if we continue to
steady the mind and heart, these states of *Samadhi* will become
more frequent and a natural ascension will occur.

All the Samadhis *described thus far have been* **Sabija** *(with*
seed), which have the ability to germinate, returning us to
ordinary consciousness.

1.47 *In the purity of* Nirvichara Samadhi, *Divine*
Consciousness becomes luminescent.

In *Nirvichara Samadhi* (perceiving knowledge of subtle forms
alone), the (karmic) seeds, while still present, are less likely to germinate. Having progressed this far, it is always possible to return to
individual consciousness, but it is less likely because of the strong
and continuous identification with the light of the Divine Self.
Each time a greater part of our consciousness remembers these

transcendental states and longs to reside in them, they become more intoxicating than our former awareness.

In the purity of Nirvichara Samadhi, *Divine Consciousness becomes luminescent.*

1.48 *When consciousness dwells in* absolute true knowledge (Ritambhara Prajna), *direct spiritual percep-tion dawns.*

1.49 *This* absolute true knowledge (Ritambhara Prajna) *is totally different from the knowledge gained by personal experience, inference, and insights from the wise.*

1.50 *When experiencing this* absolute true knowledge (Ritambhara Prajna), *all previous* Samskaras *(impressions) are left behind and new ones are prevented from sprouting.*

This absolute true knowledge (*Ritambhara Prajna*) differs from the learned knowledge described in Book I, Sutra 6. The previous knowledge derived from books, spoken words, or the senses is no longer sufficient to satisfy the deep yearning for truth.

This higher absolute true knowledge is directly imparted to us by an unseen grace. In previous stages of *Samadhi* there may be the need for guidance from our minds or hearts (i.e., stay alert, center on the object, etc.) to help us focus and maintain awareness. At this level there is a magnetic power of attraction that effortlessly draws us toward the *Ritambhara Prajna.*

When consciousness dwells in absolute true knowledge
(Ritambhara Prajna), *direct spiritual perception dawns.*

This absolute true knowledge (Ritambhara Prajna) *is totally
different from the knowledge gained by personal experience,
inference, and insights from the wise.*

When experiencing this absolute true knowledge (Ritambhara
Prajna), *all previous* Samskaras *(impressions) are left behind
and new ones are prevented from sprouting.*

1.51 Nirbija *(seedless)* Samadhi *outshines all impressions and manifestations.*

In this highest stage of. *Samadhi,* the Immortal Divine Self
shines. All the other seeds and *Samskaras* (past impressions) have
been rendered impotent. With all the *Sabija* (with seed) *Samadhis,* there is still a kernel of the subtle awareness of "I." With
Nirbija (seedless) *Samadhi,* the illusions of birth and death have
fled, and in their place is simply the knowledge of the Immortal
Divine Self.

   Living in the world in this *Samadhi,* we emanate total compassion and love, and our hearts and minds are forever united with
the one Divine Consciousness that we perceive in all. This is the
ultimate *Samadhi,* complete and everlasting Union with the
Divine.

> "Pilgrim, pilgrimage, and road—it was but myself toward my Self,
> and your arrival was but myself at my own door."
>
> —*Rumi*

Nirbija *(seedless)* Samadhi *outshines all impressions and
manifestations.*

(Please note: It is my experience that while these states of *Samadhi* are interesting to know about and can enlighten us as to the great heights we may reach, they can also veer us away from the practical. They are not states that we can *attain;* instead they are the fulfillment of our conscious evolution. My assurance to you is that, as your consciousness traverses these levels, the names and their meanings will be useless. If even for a moment your mind searches for the names or attributes of each of the *Samadhis,* you will be again back to the world of thoughts and feelings. Instead, as you visit or make a permanent residence in these exalted stages of *Samadhi,* enjoy the experience.

BOOK II.

SADHANA PADA:

Cultivation of Spiritual Practice

Book I establishes our perception that when consciousness unites we know we are Divine Beings.

Book II will reveal the practices and experiences that encourage the reunion of Consciousness.

KRIYA YOGA:
The Venerable Threefold Path

KRIYA YOGA embraces the venerable threefold path of: *Karma Yoga,* dedicated service to all; *Jnana Yoga,* intuitive wisdom; and *Bhakti Yoga,* love and devotion.

Kriya Yoga, or Yoga in Action, embraces:

Tapas: igniting the purifying flame

Swadhaya: sacred study of the Divine through scripture, nature, and introspection

Iswara Pranidhana: wholehearted dedication to the Divine Light in all.

These practices enhance inner awareness and guide us to liberation.

11.1 Kriya Yoga, or Yoga in Action, embraces:

Tapas: igniting the purifying flame

Swadhaya: sacred study of the
Divine through scripture, nature, and introspection

Iswara Pranidhana: wholehearted dedication to
the Divine Light in all.

11.2 These practices enhance inner awareness and guide us to liberation.

Kriya Yoga, or Yoga in Action, seamlessly weaves the teachings of Yoga into our everyday world, becoming a template for our hands, heads, and hearts to follow. When mixed in the correct proportions, action, thought, and feelings harmonize completely, allowing our inner spirit and the outer worlds to unite.

The practice of *Tapas* reflects *Karma Yoga* (dedicated service to all) and invites us to embrace all experiences without expecting any specific results. With this attitude, the purifying flame is ignited. The material world graciously stands ready with multiple opportunities for self-improvement and purification. The true reward is to understand and accept all challenges as gifts that enhance clarity.

Swadhaya reflects *Jnana Yoga,* encouraging us to consider and study the Divine and natural realms, and to examine ourselves just as carefully. Fine-tuning our mental and intuitive aspects, we harmonize with the inspirations that they have to offer.

Iswara Pranidhana is an aspect of *Bhakti Yoga,* the recently discussed practice of wholehearted dedication to the Divine Light in all. Through this practice, the intoxication of the Divine is made present at every moment and with every action.

"The hand stays in society while the heart rests with the Divine"
—*Bhagavad-Gita*

This is a mighty and blessed formula.

THE GODDESS GAYATRI BREATHES LIFE INTO THE WORLD

The same triad of power present in *Kriya Yoga* is reflected most simply in the ancient *Gayatri Mantra*. This Sacred Mantra is the Universal Prayer enshrined in the *Rig Veda*. Chanted for thousands of years, it invokes the Divine Light, honored through the ages as the source of our continued creation. By dedicated repetition of *Gayatri,* all the wisdom and practices of *Kriya Yoga* can be experienced.

The sacred prayer is dedicated to the goddess Gayatri, a feminine aspect of pure consciousness who is considered to be the Mother of the *Vedas*. From Divine Light, she creates all life. She resides within the heart of human souls as she outwardly enhances the splendor of the natural world.

Until recently this mantra has been kept in strict secrecy. Only those purified by initiation were permitted to hear this sacred prayer, let alone chant it, as they yearned for its dynamic power of liberation.

The goddess Gayatri in her compassion has recently offered this transformational mantra to the uninitiated secular world. Its powerful and purifying effects permeate all environments, affecting the entire globe on profound levels. Chanting along to a recording of *Gayatri Mantra,* or even just listening to it, one readily experiences its power.

The sacred *Gayatri Mantra* is a unique way to understand *Kriya Yoga*. It deepens spiritual understanding without the intervention of the mind. Repetition of the mantra channels its vibratory meaning directly to the heart.

Om Bhur Bhuvah Swaha
Tat savitur varenyam
Bhargo devasya dhimahi
Dhiyo yonah prachodayat.

Embracing Earth, Heaven and Beyond
The sacred source is revealed
Evoking the resplendent flame
The all-pervading light venerates us all.

Kriya Yoga, *or Yoga in Action, embraces*
Swadhaya: *sacred study of the Divine through scripture,*
nature, and introspection

From Gayatri
  Om Bhur Bhuvah Swaha / Tat savitur varenyam
  Embracing Earth, Heaven and Beyond / The sacred
    source is revealed

The first two lines of the *Gayatri Mantra* represent reflective study on all three levels encased in the Divine and natural realms, and this relates to *Swadhaya.* *Bhur* refers to the earth, *Bhuva* the heavens, and *Swaha* (notice the *swa* is also the first part of *Swadhaya*) the higher consciousness beyond the worlds we know. With study we are able to ascend to the highest level, to the source we hold sacred.

TO STUDY IS TO LOVE

Swadhaya study comes in many forms. To aid in our worldly and Divine studies, we are blessed to have an extensive range of books available to us. With that availability comes the responsibility to cultivate a high level of discrimination. Adapting study as a spiritual practice addresses our social responsibility as well as that of our intellect.

As Parmahansa Yogandanda once said, "Read a sentence from a book and when you have incorporated it into your life go on to the next sentence." This great quote gives us a glimpse into the quality of study we are seeking as well as the devotion and dedication necessary. Evaluate the books you are reading. Are your books stimulating your consciousness, inspiring you to do great things? Or are they just inspiring dust to collect? Better to have a few choice books that encourage you than a huge library that clutters your shelves and your mind. Books can be great teachers when they encourage us to take the high road and bestow compassion on others. Many people still read and adhere to the time-honored classics because, in one form or another, they pass on this gem of wisdom.

Swadhaya also encourages study of the natural world by observing with awe her bounty and the uniqueness of everyday life. Greet the morning light with reverence and wonder, and with the diminishing light welcome the miracle of night as you draw inward. Let each butterfly and ant have a delightful presence in your life. Study nature and feel the comfort of her presence.

Children are our best teachers for studying nature. Ever take a walk with a three- or four-year-old? You might have said something like, "Come on, honey, we can't stop and look at every little bug!" Instead of teaching our children to hurry, let the babes teach us to marvel at nature.

Kriya Yoga, *or Yoga in Action, embraces*
   Swadhaya: *sacred study of the Divine through scripture, nature, and introspection*

   From Gayatri
      Om Bhur Bhuvah Swaha / Tat savitur varenyam
      Embracing Earth, Heaven and Beyond / The sacred source is revealed

When we embark on a journey of introspection or a deep study on ourselves, we tend to see the surface of our bodies and recognize the shortcomings. Perhaps we notice a few more wrinkles, another gray hair, that chocolate éclair that went straight to the hips. How different we would feel if we took the time to really look at the miracle of life and repeat a gentle phrase or affirmation, a smile of recognition. Remind yourself constantly that you are a Divine Being, nothing more, nothing less, and nothing else! To know and love the higher aspect of yourself is an exquisite way to practice *Swadhaya*.

THE SEED OF THE UNIVERSE

Within the aspect of *Swadhaya* are prayer and *japa* (repetition of a mantra).

A mantra is a one- or many-syllable sound that transcends the mind and emotions. If repeated for its vibrational effect, it brings us to the level of *Swaha*. A mantra is like a seed: its simplicity hides the potential power it holds. Seeing a tiny acorn, it is difficult to imagine the mighty oak tree within. Likewise, though it might not seem like much, the smallest mantra (like *"Om"*), when repeated with the heart, has the power to unite us with our Divine nature.

Swadhaya: *sacred study of the Divine through scripture, nature, and introspection*
   Om Bhur Bhuvah Swaha / Tat savitur varenyam
   Embracing Earth, Heaven and Beyond / The sacred source is revealed

Kriya Yoga, *or Yoga in Action, embraces*
   Tapas: *igniting the purifying flame*

From Gayatri
  Bhargo devasya dhimahi . . .
  Evoking the resplendent flame

Tapas is taken literally to mean burn or purify. In a higher sense it is an attitude that allows us to embrace all of life's experiences as a means for purification, be they pleasant or unpleasant.

A truckload of gold ore would appear to most of us as a bunch of ordinary black rocks. To be purified, the ore is heaved into a scalding hot fire. The impurities slowly turn to ash, leaving a minute quantity of sparkling purified gold (alchemy at play). Gold's worth is measured by its purity, so the longer it remains in the fire, the more refined—and more valuable—it becomes. First it becomes 12 karats, then 14, and, with continued firing, the purest and most precious 24-karat gold emerges.

For most traditions this kind of refinement is made available to our consciousness through *Karma Yoga,* the path of selfless service, the alchemy that purifies the heart and mind. Often in the name of spiritual growth, *tapas* will be interpreted as asceticism. This is an unfortunate euphemism for overworking or even harming the body, mind, and emotions. In an effort to "detach" from the "pleasures" of the body, people are known to fast for prolonged periods of time, stand on one leg for days, lie on beds of nails, walk on hot coals, wear hair shirts, and partake in any number of practices to induce pain. They think that anything that magnifies discomfort will surely burn away impurities and control the mind! Often, though, the opposite occurs as the body and mind cry out for comfort and relief. Many of these austerities can also seriously damage the body, defacing the temple that houses the Divine spirit.

"Those who seek to destroy the body, also destroy me, the indweller."
—*Bhagavad-Gita*

Although outwardly very spectacular, these austerities are *not* the highest form of *Tapas*. Conjuring up any form of *Tapas* is not really necessary, as it seems that with each new day the world serves up new challenges by which we are purified. If we intentionally add discomfort or pain to an already weakened body or mind, this tends to further separate us from the Divine spirit. Pay close attention in your own life to how *Tapas* manifests. Its hardships may even persuade you to doubt the existence of the Divine—but in the end, see if you aren't purified by its flames.

Kriya Yoga, *or Yoga in Action, embraces*
    Tapas: *igniting the purifying flame*

From Gayatri
    Bhargo devasya dhimahi . . .
    Evoking the resplendent flame

THE OPPORTUNITIES FOR *TAPAS* ARE UNLIMITED

Imagine you have been driving around looking for parking and, just as you are backing into a space, someone barges in and takes it. Or maybe you are on the freeway and a car cuts in front of you, causing you to brake quickly. Can you avoid shuttling that anger and frustration onto yourself or those around you? Are you able to embrace these emotions and inconveniences as a means for purification, or do they give you a good excuse to curse and shout?

What if it is not a human disturbance but an external one, like a dead car battery? The car is already packed; you are ready to embark on a much-needed weekend away. Your route is mapped out to miss the stream of traffic on Friday night. You turn the ignition and nothing happens! The idea of missing the traffic and getting to your destination before dark is completely lost. Do you see it as a wonderful time to manage the frustration you are holding in the mind and emotions, or is it an excuse to scream at the next person who detains you? How we react to these situations becomes the framework of our spiritual practice.

Even the most minute of disturbances during our formal Yoga practices can send us plummeting from the higher realms back to the material world. A tiny mosquito buzzing in your ear during deep relaxation can quickly turn the practice into an arm-waving event worthy of Olympic competition. If, though, we use *Tapas* to tether ourselves close to our center, its transcendent power moves with us into daily life.

The more luminescent we are, the more we are able to serve without wanting rewards. If an unpleasant situation should occur, we accept it as a means for purification, returning only joy and love. This is considered one of the best and most challenging forms of *Tapas*. The supreme purpose of *Tapas* is to accept life's challenges while being loving and compassionate to all, especially ourselves.

At times it might feel as if we are doled a greater portion of *Tapas* than we can handle. Those are the times to draw upon the strength we have gained from the formal practices, and to be grateful for it (if we can).

Mother Teresa of Calcutta was asked during a moment of great trial if she thought Jesus ever tested her beyond her limits. She hesitated slightly before she responded: "No, I don't think I am ever tested beyond my limits, but I often wish He did not have such a high opinion of me!"

Kriya Yoga, *or Yoga in Action, embraces*
Tapas: *igniting the purifying flame*

From Gayatri
    Bhargo devasya dhimahi . . .
    Evoking the resplendent flame

Kriya Yoga, *or Yoga in Action, embraces*
  Iswara Pranidhana: *wholehearted dedication to the Divine
  Light in all*

  From Gayatri
    Dhiyo yonah prachodayat.
    The all-pervading light venerates us all.

Iswara Pranidhana is a recurrent theme throughout the sutras. It
is often considered one of the most pleasing and among the easiest
of practices.

By sprinkling life with devotion, each and every moment of it
can be transformed. Our ultimate awakening may come simply by
pausing regularly to feel this wholehearted dedication to the
all-pervading light within.

The human mind has difficulty comprehending something as vast
as an all-pervading omniscient consciousness. Throughout its his-
tory, human society has narcissistically associated its own image with
that of the Divine. Further evolution of this concept projected a
human *male* likeness onto the formless, solidifying the exclusivity of
male divinity. The writers and translators, almost exclusively men
themselves, endorsed this characterization. Up until very recently,
the masculine nature of the Divine was an undisputed reality.

As women, our experience of the Divine energy is often found in
communion with the changing cycles of nature, in the joys we reap
from our personal relationships, in the love of our families. Our dedication and devotion, while easily expressed, is often unrecipro-
cated. Frequently, in the search for returned affection, we lavish our
wholehearted devotion on one or more masculine images (fathers,
sons, husbands, ministers, priests, rabbis, teachers, etc.), ignoring
the Divine within ourselves. We need to discover ways to value our
own power even as our hearts remain entwined with others.

By delving into our hearts, we pass the boundaries of our limited
minds and recognize the Divine Consciousness as primordial

energy within each living thing. A person, an animal, a falling leaf, or a sinking stone—all are part of the Divine. When we make this realization with our hearts, we are drawn in love to the Divine energy in all things, and the whole world becomes our beloved. How could it really be otherwise?

Kriya Yoga, *or Yoga in Action, embraces:*
Iswara Pranidhana: *wholehearted dedication to the Divine Light in all*

From Gayatri
 Dhiyo yonah prachodayat.
 The all-pervading light venerates us all.

EXPERIENCING *KRIYA YOGA* THROUGH CHANTING OF THE *GAYATRI MANTRA*

Learn and begin to repeat the Gayatri Mantra *a few times a day.*

As you hear the Sanskrit, remind yourself of the translation in English. Understand and experience the words as their truth resonates in your heart.

 Om Bhur Bhuvah Swaha
 Tat savitur varenyam
 Bhargo devasya dhimahi
 Dhiyo yonah prachodayat.

Embracing Earth, Heaven, and Beyond
The sacred source is revealed [reflecting Swadhaya]
Evoking the resplendent flame [reflecting Tapas]
The all-pervading light venerates us all [reflecting Iswara Pranidhana].

After a time, let go of the literal meaning and just focus on the vibration. Notice how it resonates in your heart, reverberating through your body, thoughts, and emotions, glazing your entire life. (If this is an unfamiliar chant, you can purchase one of the many CDs available. Find one with a tune that resonates with your heart and is easy to chant along with.)

After the formal sitting, enjoy the Gayatri Mantra *playing in the background while you work or play. The meaning will continue to vibrate within your heart.*

EXPERIENCING *KRIYA* YOGA IN EVERYDAY LIFE

Observe the different aspects of Kriya Yoga *and how you've practiced them throughout the day.*

Create a practice for each of the three aspects of Kriya Yoga *that is meaningful to you. Change or alter the practices as you choose.*

What would your practice of Karma Yoga *(Selfless Service) and* Tapas *(igniting the purifying flame) be like?*

What would your practice of Jnana Yoga *(intuitive wisdom) and* Swadhaya *(sacred study of the Divine) be like?*

What would your practice of Bhakti Yoga *(devotion) and* Iswara Pranidhana *(wholehearted dedication to the Divine Light in all) be like?*

Allow all three to dance together in your life, bringing you to wholeness.

THE *KLESHAS:* *Dissolving the Veils*

THERE ARE FIVE veils that cover the light of the Divine Self, obscuring it from recognition. When we become aware of them, the veils dissolve one by one, and the Divine Light within is seen again.

Dissolving the five Kleshas, or veils, brings forth the radiance of the Divine Self.

The five Kleshas, or veils, are:
Avidya: innocence of our Divine nature
Asmita: undue trust in the individual self
Raga: excessive fondness of fleeting pleasures
Dvesa: excessive avoidance of unpleasant experiences
Abhinivesah: elusive awareness of immortality.

Innocence of our Divine nature (Avidya) creates a fertile field where the dormant seeds of the other four veils take root.

Innocence of our Divine nature (Avidya) encourages identification with the ever changing, rather than with the inner stillness of the heart.

When undue trust is placed in the individual self (Asmita), it is confused with the Divine Self.

Excessive fondness for fleeting pleasures (Raga)
causes longing.

Excessive avoidance of unpleasant experiences (Dvesa)
causes disdain.

*The elusive awareness of immortality is inherent even
for the wise* (Abhinivesah).

With keen observation and discretion, these Kleshas
become translucent.

*If they have manifested into action, the veils must be
dissolved through inward practice.*

11.3 *Dissolving the five* Kleshas, *or veils, brings forth the radiance of the* Divine Self.

> *The five* Kleshas, *or veils, are:*
> Avidya: *innocence of our Divine nature*
> Asmita: *undue trust in the individual self*
> Raga: *excessive fondness of fleeting pleasures*
> Dvesa: *excessive avoidance of unpleasant experiences*
> Abhinivesah: *elusive awareness of immortality.*

The Divine within is self-effulgent. With the donning of a physical body at birth, certain mental and emotional beliefs materialize as veils. At first these veils are translucent, and the radiant light still shines through. When we look into the eyes of a newborn baby, they reflect the clarity of the resplendent light. As we become increasingly invested in the material world, the seeds of infinite possibilities for wonderful or unkind actions encased in the mind and emotions germinate. The veils thicken and the knowledge that we are Divine Beings fades.

We falsely adopt our fleeting thoughts and emotions as our identity, further occluding the light within. We lose even the memory of its radiance. The belief that we are "merely human" has become our truth.

KEEP THE LIGHT SHINING BRIGHTLY

Did you ever use a kerosene lamp? At first the light shines bright, illuminating the darkness, enabling us to see clearly. After some time, the glass chimney begins to blacken with soot and the light dims. Turning up the flame only causes the soot to thicken, until the light is totally obscured. Reluctant to clean it earlier, we become obliged to remove the chimney, wash it, and replace it. The yogic practices dissolve the veils in a process similar to cleaning the chimney. With this new clarity, the light shines clear and bright.

Dissolving the five Kleshas, or veils, brings forth the radiance of the Divine Self.

11.4 *Innocence of our Divine nature* (Avidya) *creates a fertile field where the dormant seeds of the other four veils take root.*

As the veil of innocence envelops our Divine nature, the environment becomes conducive for the other four veils to deeply root. When this essential veil lifts, we behold our Divine nature, and the other four veils become powerless.

11.5 *Innocence of our Divine nature* (Avidya) *encourages identification with the ever changing, rather than with the inner stillness of the heart.*

Our lives, hopes, and dreams are built with the conviction that we have some influence over the forces of nature. Often those same hopes and dreams evaporate with the first change in the wind. These changes keep our minds reeling, our hearts in constant hope, and our dreams just out of reach. If we are fortunate enough to realize our dreams, we may after a short time become bored with them as the next castle in the sky forms in our imagination. These dreams are like snowflakes, melting as soon as we take hold of them. Yet day after day we continue to accept triumphs and disappointments as an integral part of the ever-changing nature.

When we turn our view inward, a grand discovery awaits us. Here we find a sacred place where stillness and peace abide, encouraging our hearts to blossom.

This concept is elegantly portrayed in the spiritual practice of turning or whirling practiced by the mystical Middle Eastern order of Sufism. The great Sufi mystic and poet Mevlana Rumi founded the Whirling Dervishes. Enraptured by the dance of life, the ceremonial turning and whirling inspires even the unbeliever. Arms outstretched in surrender, the left palm pays homage to the earth, the right to heaven. While the left foot is rooted to the world, the right pulses up and down rhythmically to the heart's prayer. The grace and indrawn attention is present in the elegant circular movements. The dance mimics life as the union of constant movement and stillness; all the while the heart stays entwined with the Divine.

Recognizing the Divine within, we dance through the world with joy.

Innocence of our Divine nature (Avidya) encourages identification with the ever changing, rather than with the inner stillness of the heart.

11.6 *When undue trust is placed in the individual self (Asmita), it is confused with the Divine Self.*

Even in the most extraordinary events, the Divine remains anonymous. We accept praise and credit for most of the things we do: "*I* built that"; "*I* healed that person." Do you really believe that you, as an individual self, have the capacity to build something of extraordinary beauty or that you hold the power to heal? This narrow vision of our interaction with the physical world may help to build individual self-esteem, but it fails to capture the ultimate reality.

What happens if your accomplishment is challenged or criticized? Often we become overly upset, terrified to try again.

If, instead, your sense of self-esteem is based on the belief that you are Divine, then you will know that all your actions come from that source. Living this way, you will always feel connected to the cosmic dance.

A wise friend reminded me that there were three important words to remember: "No," "Yes," and "Wow." Try using them in the quantity that the order represents. Use "No" sparingly. It will allow you to have a certain illusory control over your life, but in excess it breeds resistance, fear, and even anger. Overuse of "No" promotes a heaviness and rigidity in your life.

A generous sprinkling of "Yes" throughout your life encourages openness and adventure as it leaves the door open for new possibilities. "Yes" also encourages us to surrender the idea of control and let the heart take over. Life is never dull when you use "Yes" frequently.

Saying and thinking "Wow" as much as possible will inspire a sense of wonder and gratitude, reminding you of the infinite potential of the Divine Self.

When undue trust is placed in the individual self (**Asmita**), **it is confused with the Divine Self.**

II.7 *Excessive fondness for fleeting pleasures* (Raga) *causes longing.*

II.8 *Excessive avoidance of unpleasant experiences* (Dvesa) *causes disdain.*

These sutras represent the extremes of the swinging pendulum that tend to overshadow our lives: good and evil, pleasure and pain, love and hate. We tend to think toward the extremes. Actually, there are infinite possibilities between them. Realizing this, we can stop at any one of the midway points and find balance and comfort there. Our hope in practicing Yoga is that our life will stabilize in this way.

Continually striving for the highs, we will probably find that they elude us, and we will feel compelled to climb to steeper and steeper plateaus. We enjoy the thrill of the highest mountain, but dislike roaming around in the endless valleys below. Instead, we could be seeking out the endless plain of harmony.

BUT DID THEY LIVE HAPPILY EVER AFTER?

Having been a monk and a spiritual minister for many years, I find that one of the joys of this vocation is presiding over weddings. On that magical day, each pledges love and dedication to the other. My heart never fails to delight in the splendor of love.

For a growing majority of couples, something changes after the earnestness of the vows. On their wedding day, they've promised to cling to each other for richer or for poorer, in sickness and in health, forsaking all others. Fast-forward several years, and the same two lovebirds have turned into birds of prey. They stand together not at a spiritual altar, but at the bar of a court of law. The passion that once fanned the flames of love now swirls the fire of animosity, fueled by wounded feelings and accusations. I often wonder, "What could have caused such a dramatic change?"

If we are used to extremes, we may find ourselves bored when balance and calm come to prevail. When falling in love, at the peak of great passion, it is difficult to remember that there is a valley deep below. Instead of scaling the peaks only to fly off a cliff, ride the peaceful, rolling hills. A balanced relationship promotes growth and liberation for all involved.

Excessive fondness for fleeting pleasures (Raga) *causes longing.*

Excessive avoidance of unpleasant experiences (Dvesa) *causes disdain.*

The *Bhagavad-Gita* counsels us on the virtues of the middle path: "Peace is granted to those who see the same Self in friend and foe alike, whose mind stays balanced in the midst of honor or dishonor, heat or cold, pleasure or pain, and who maintains equanimity during praise and blame."

The *Gita* is not advocating avoidance or overindulgence; rather, it points to the mystical path of balance. Often in our zeal for spiritual practices, we feel it is essential to become an ascetic, eliminating the pleasures of the physical world. But in eliminating all the little niceties that make life on the earth fun and enjoyable, we are looking for divinity externally, and risk forgetting that what we are seeking is already within us.

SWEETS MAKE US SWEET

While in India I had the great blessing of being invited to an intimate *satsang* (company of the wise) with Sri Shastraji, a great Yoga Master. As he spoke about the *Vedas* and other such elevated subjects, a plate of tasty treats was placed in front of him. Continuing his discourse, he offered the sweets, encouraging me to take as many as I would like.

He must have noticed my beaming smile as I reached for more than a few. "Ah," he said, "you like sweets?"

"I love sweets!" I said. The great philosopher asked me why.

"Well," I thought for a moment, reluctantly taking my attention away from the taste sensation in my mouth, "they make me sweet!"

"What a great understanding of the teachings." He chuckled. "The *Vedas* tell us that when we are able to experience the *sukha* [sweetness or happiness] of life in any form, it serves to remind us of the Divine Self. If we do not experience sweetness, we assume that it is not there. With the absence of *sukha,* our only option is to identify with the opposite, *dukha* [sadness or bitterness]."

Many teachers and translators of the scriptures encourage us to avoid the sweetness in life to better prepare us for the big payoff, *enlightenment.* It is actually the opposite. By generously sprinkling our lives with joy and sweetness, their seeds take root within us, reflecting in our every action. This ever-present joy is the greatest enlightenment and it can be ours right now!

Excessive fondness for fleeting pleasures (Raga) *causes longing.*

Excessive avoidance of unpleasant experiences (Dvesa) *causes disdain.*

II.9 *The elusive awareness of immortality is inherent even for the wise* (Abhinivesah).

One of the most vital reasons for spiritual practice is to prepare us for the moment of physical death. Dying can be a time when great apprehension and doubt become our constant companions. Remembering that we are Divine and therefore immortal can ease that struggle.

The more we busy ourselves with life's diversions, the less we identify with our bodies' constant wear and tear. Yet our breath betrays us by continuing to count down our allotted time. People diagnosed with life-threatening diseases often have a keener awareness of the "now." They have the grace to know their fate and decide priorities based on a limited engagement on this precious earth. Sometimes it seems their lust for life is stronger than most of ours is, since we delude ourselves into thinking we have an unlimited, noncancelable contract.

The curious way we think of life and death in our society is carved on each gravestone.

NAME
BORN–DIED
1908–2000

How do you interpret this information? Both dates are very important, the first being when she was born into this world, and the second when she left this world. And the dash? That was the rest of her life! A dash, interesting! It is as if we are born, and we begin to dash to our goal—death. After ninety-two years of running, it seems she finally made it!

We need a reminder *not* to dash. Instead, slow down and appreciate each moment for its beauty and fullness.

The elusive awareness of immortality is inherent even for the wise (**Abhinivesah**).

A SAINT FOR ALL REASONS

My foremost inspiration from a saintly woman came in the form of Sri Sharada Devi. Most commonly known as the wife of Sri Ramakrishna Paramahansa, she was a Luminous Teacher in her own right, known to many as the Holy Mother. In her humility the Holy Mother expressed the teachings through her living example.

Often friends or students coming to me during a life crisis did not want to express their emotions, fearing I would find them lacking in "spirituality." In an endeavor to comfort them, I often related one of my favorite teachings from Sri Sharada Devi.

After the death of Sri Ramakrishna, the Holy Mother became

the spiritual head (better yet, the spiritual heart!) of the organization. In spite of the fact that the master himself honored her with the position, some of the male monastic disciples doubted that a *woman* could have the spiritual attainment to advise them.

There were, however, a few who recognized her divinity. One young monk who revered her as the Divine Mother personally attended to her needs and served her food with love, devotion, and reverence.

She expected him this particular morning, when another monk appeared with her breakfast. "Where," she asked, "is my *other* dear son?"

"Mother," replied the monk, "I am here to inform you that in the night he left his mortal coil." Immediately on hearing this, tears cascaded down her cheeks. Abandoning herself to grief, she began to sob.

"Mother, how can *you* resort to such emotion? You know that the body is just temporary, that only the soul is immortal. *We are not the body or the mind!*" He had the gall to quote *Vedanta* (scripture) to her!

With a compassionate smile emanating from her pure heart, she said, "Yes, my son, I know all the sacred teachings. Yet I am still in human form and, therefore, have feelings. Right now my heart is breaking for the physical loss of my beloved son. I honor that pain with my tears."

Within the spiritual traditions, both mind and heart must be honored. Since much emphasis is placed on controlling the mind, it is vital to give the heart its place of honor. It is the guardian to the spark of divinity, the True Self. Be joyful and remember your own immortality.

> "I died a mineral and became a plant. I died a plant and rose as an animal. I died an animal and I was man (or woman). Why should I fear? When was I less by dying?"
>
> —*Rumi*

The elusive awareness of immortality is inherent even for the wise (Abhinivesah).

ii.10 *With keen observation and discretion, these Kleshas become translucent.*

If the veils are present in *feeling and thought,* keen observation is enough to enable us to disperse them.

With keen observation and discretion, these Kleshas *become* translucent.

ii.11 *If they have manifested into action, the veils must be dissolved through inward practice.*

When the *Kleshas* manifest in words and actions, their roots are already deep. Mere observation is not enough to displace them. This is the time to call upon the deeper, subtler, and therefore more powerful inner practices. Periods of stillness, introspection, and devotion are summoned to dissolve the veils that hide the inner light.

If they have manifested into action, the veils must be dissolved through inward practice.

EXPERIENCING THE DISSOLVING
OF THE FIVE *KLESHAS*

Find a comfortable position, either lying down on the floor or on your bed.

Place your right hand on your lower belly and your left hand on your heart.

Begin to observe your breath. Is it deep and regular? Shallow and irregular?

Shift your attention to the idea that breath propels life.

Each time you inhale, there is an inflow of life's energy entering your body.

With the exhalation observe the energy leaving your body.

This is followed by a moment's hesitation, a space between the two breaths and between the two worlds.

Notice any discomfort in your body, emotions, or mind.

Continue for a few minutes. Invoke the attitude of gratitude for this life-giving breath.

Now, gradually, shift your attention to the center of your heart and the light that dwells within, the Divine Self.

Can you begin to experience the light of the Divine Self?

Be still and patient until you feel the veils thinning.

Can you identify any aspect of your belief system that keeps the veil of innocence (Avidya) in place?

Once you have identified it, can you envision a symbol, a feeling, or a word that can return you to the light of the Divine?

Breathe deeply, enhancing the energy and spreading the light through the body, mind, and emotions, coming back to full consciousness.

Tuck the memory of this experience deep into the recesses of your heart and sprinkle it liberally throughout your day.

After some time, and with continuous practice, you will find the veils become more and more transparent.

As the Divine Light radiates through us, it illuminates who we are, shedding light on all we do.

CHAPTER

3

KARMA AND *KARMA YOGA:*
As You Sow, So You Shall Reap

THESE SUTRAS ATTEMPT to explain the intricate aspects of karma, the cycle of actions seeding other actions. Its concept is widely known, and often quite misunderstood. Hopefully, this commentary will alleviate some of the confusion and allow you to understand the basic principles and intent of karma.

The womb of karma (Karmasala), sheathed by the Kleshas (veils), gives birth to experiences now and in the future.

As long as the veils encase the womb of karma (Karmasala), all actions will be affected.

Karma bears fruits according to the type and quality of the seed planted, and the care given to its growth.

II.12 *The womb of karma* (Karmasala), *sheathed by the* Kleshas *(veils), gives birth to experiences now and in the future.*

II.13 *As long as the veils encase the womb of karma* (Karmasala), *all actions will be affected.*

II.14 *Karma bears fruits according to the type and quality of the seed planted, and the care given to its growth.*

"Karma" is popularly understood as a kind of universal punishment for our sins and a reward for our good deeds. This simplistic definition is reinforced by the notion of someone or something far above us passing judgment and sentencing us. So when bad things happen to good people, we are outraged at the unfairness of life and question the sanity of this higher judge.

The concept of karma depicted in the *Yoga Sutras* and the *Bhagavad-Gita* is in fact a neutral energy that when activated by the mind and emotions, manifests into action. This action leads to a reaction that in turn spawns new action and continues the cycle. It is our choice, though not always a conscious one, whether to move karma into fruition or let it remain dormant. While most of us choose to believe that the actions of others have the greatest effect on us, it is actually our own deeds that have the most profound influence.

The idea of blame or judgment is removed if we understand that our karma is directly affected by the density of the veils *(Kleshas)* that cloak our Divine nature. When filtered through opaque layers, the inner light appears dim and distorted. This significantly alters our motives and our actions. Unable to easily identify with our true nature, we think and act for material gain. This is what turns the constant spinning wheel of action and reaction that drives us day after day, month after month, life after life.

Looking at the world from a dualistic view, we eagerly polarize karma into good or bad, white or black. Instead, when we view it as a rainbow of colors, each karma brings us a message to shape our lives.

Karma is similar to the energy of an electrical current. The outlet in your house supplies needed electricity. Is that good or bad? If you plug in a lamp and receive light, you might say, "Ah! Electricity is good. I have good karma; there is light to read at night." However, if you stick your finger into that same outlet and get a shock, you might think, "Ah! Electricity is bad! What bad karma I must have to get shocked in my own home." Electricity, like karma, is neither good nor bad; its affect is determined by how we treat it.

Individual karmas become our teachers, encouraging us to remember the True Self. When a few join together for a larger lesson, the consequences often seem disproportionate to the minor event that gave birth to them. It is those times that reinforce our belief that karma is either bad or good. In fact, it is just a bigger lesson for us to learn.

THE FRUITS RIPEN IN THREE WAYS

Managing our karma is like planting and tending a garden. Before planting any garden, we first must realistically consider what plants grow well in the particular soil and climate. Each plant or tree, depending on the conditions, has the potential to produce delicious fruits or inedible ones. We must use our best judgment as to which seeds to plant and which plants to nourish.

Three types of karma emerge from the womb of karma (*Karmasala*) into our garden: *Agami, Parabda,* and *Sangita.*

Agami is the karma that governs those actions that are already determined and cannot be changed, such as where and when you were born, who your birth parents are, and so on. You may wish you could change these events, but it is not possible. The trees planted long before are now bearing fruit. It is too late to change the type of fruit *or* the taste.

Parabda karma gives us time to make changes, but only if we act promptly. Careful consideration must be taken before planting. Having prepared the soil and gathered seedlings from a sweet apple, we lovingly place them in the earth. We know that we will be rewarded with a great harvest if each plant receives the optimum amount of water, sun, and room to grow. We carefully eliminate those plants that spring up to threaten the delicate seedlings. When we plant and weed with discrimination and compassion, the plants we are caring for will thrive. Likewise, the karmas we are planting now bear fruit in the future.

If we plant a peach seed, it would be unrealistic to expect to come back after a few years and pick apples. If at the time of planting, the seeds were inferior, or the tree was not well tended, the fruit will reflect those conditions. We may not be able to change the quality of the fruits; we can, however, change our attitude toward them. Instead of chiding a tree for producing sour apples, the creative solution would be to add a little sweetener and make an apple pie!

You might have heard a friend say something to this effect: "My fiancé is not very kind to me. Maybe *after* we get married, his attitude will change." Expecting someone to change is a dangerous notion. This is the time to nip *Parabda* karma in the bud. A well-considered decision not to marry this person can eliminate heartache in the future.

Sangita karma keeps the seeds safe within the *Karmasala*. They are yet unsprouted. Assessing whether to plant the seeds of karma, we recall certain life experiences and plant with caution, knowing that once the seeds germinate, we reap the harvest. Even if we try to pull them up, the roots have grown deep, and the underground growth may continue. It is best to honor our intuition regarding which of the incubating seeds we plant.

Your choices may sound something like this. "This situation reminds me of the time I stayed in that job because it paid well even though it made me miserable. Now that a similar situation has come up, I was almost fooled into doing the same thing again. But I caught myself in time."

We are not alone in our karma. Each person we meet has some influence on how our karma plays out. When you are single, your karma is entwined with that of your friends and family. If you marry, you now have your karma, his karma, and your combined karma, not to mention children, in-laws, grandchildren, and so many others. The winds of change scatter our karmic seeds far and wide.

Innumerable seeds from this life and previous ones are housed in the *Karmasala,* and it may seem that many of them come to fruition at once. We have accumulated needs for action or reaction—karmas—from all our choices in this life. If this seems overwhelming, it may be helpful to stretch our concept of mortality to understand that we, as souls, will incarnate many times to fulfill the many karmas.

The womb of karma (Karmasala), *sheathed by the* Kleshas (veils), *gives birth to experiences now and in the future.*

As long as the veils encase the womb of karma (Karmasala), *all actions will be affected.*

Karma bears fruits according to the type and quality of the seed planted, and the care given to its growth.

HOW THE *GUNAS* (ATTRIBUTES OF NATURE) INTERPLAY WITH KARMA

> "No one is free of action (karma) even for a moment because
> each is helplessly moved by the *gunas*."
>
> —*Bhagavad-Gita*

The ever-present *gunas* (attributes of nature) are forces that influence not only our karma but also our attitude toward it. If we are able to recognize and transcend the *gunas*, karma will be affected less.

Enmeshed in the *Tamasic,* or static, *guna,* we may be blind to the cause of our circumstances. We hold the attitude then that we can do anything we want without suffering the consequences. This blindness can inadvertently create more karma.

A teenager's wild driving is spurred on by her inability to imagine losing control of the tremendous machine she is manipulating. A benign near-miss might cause her arrogance to retreat, but a boomerang effect can cause the *Tamas* to deepen, presenting fear and immobility. The balance point of *Sattwa* is not even in view.

If we are steeped in the *Rajasic guna,* we are constantly irritated by how unfair life is, believing we deserve better. Sometimes, gloating when good things happen to us, we ignore the circumstances or feelings of others. When we are immersed in *Rajas,* we tend to not share our good fortune, and this brings more karma upon us.

When overly *Rajasic* people are diagnosed with a disease, they may become upset and feel victimized. This anger, diverted into righteous indignation, can prompt them to speak out against the unfair health-care system, or they may start a class-action suit against a company for misleading the public. These actions may not eradicate their karma on the disease level, but certainly can help them and others not to create any more karma in this arena.

"A moment's hesitation in anger will save a hundred days of sorrow."

—*Chinese proverb*

When we abide predominately with the *Sattwic guna,* we accept any and all karmas that come with equanimity, realizing they are blessings in disguise. If, unexpectedly, we were to receive a large amount of money, our immediate response would be to share it with those in need. When negative circumstances befall us, we understand it comes from seeds planted long before. Acceptance allows us to soothe the reaction to this karma, thwarting any need to make others suffer. We can feel that, by contributing to another's pain, we are not relieved; instead, our own suffering intensifies. With the grace of compassion, we understand the suffering of others. If we are able to metaphorically "walk a mile in another's moccasins," we may actually feel blessed by our karma.

Whenever someone complained about life's woes, my mother would say, "Take your troubles and put them in the center of a circle with all the other troubles in the world. Examine them all. I bet you will be grateful to choose yours once again."

The womb of karma (Karmasala), *sheathed by the* Kleshas (*veils*), *gives birth to experiences now and in the future.*

As long as the veils encase the womb of karma (Karmasala), *all actions will be affected.*

Karma bears fruits according to the type and quality of the seed planted, and the care given to its growth.

TRANSFORMING KARMA

Looking through the teachings of the Old and New Testaments we find karma apparent in many sections. One of the most notable is "an eye for an eye and a tooth for a tooth." It seems that thousands of years later we are still battling, plotting our revenge, or trying to get even with something or someone, making it our duty not to let anyone get away with anything.

Asked about the adage, the Reverend Martin Luther King Jr. mused, "If we follow the words of the Old Testament *exactly,* and take an eye for an eye and a tooth for a tooth, we will all become *blind and toothless."*

Constantly plagued by the mounting annoyances of everyday life, we are able to use the myriad Yoga practices to connect with the *Sattwic* aspect of our nature. Challenging as it might be, after some time the mind and emotions will acquiesce to calmness rather than aggravation.

> "Whatever greatness a person does is followed by others who set their values by her/his example. They will not disturb others who may be still attached to the fruits of their actions. By continuously performing selfless actions, the wise person influences others in all they do."
> —*Bhagavad-Gita*

The womb of karma (Karmasala), *sheathed by the* Kleshas (veils), *gives birth to experiences now and in the future.*

As long as the veils encase the womb of karma (Karmasala), *all actions will be affected.*

Karma bears fruits according to the type and quality of the seed planted, and the care given to its growth.

TRANSFORMING KARMA THROUGH *KARMA YOGA*

If action is inevitable, how can we circumvent the need for reaction and prevent more karma from accruing? Can we slow down the ever-spinning wheel? The secret is *Karma Yoga* or *Seva* (Selfless Service).

Karma Yoga tempers the law of karma (action and its subsequent reaction) by redirecting the effects of our actions through selfless service. If we must reap what we sow, let us sow seeds of a sweet and tasty fruit.

There are as many ways to serve as people to be served. *Karma Yoga* is about doing our best, not expecting praise or blame. To do the deed for the sake of doing, not looking for the reward, is at the heart of *Karma Yoga*. We may feel gratified in seeing others happy, but let this be a side effect, not the main goal.

> "One thing I know: The only ones among you who will be really happy are those who will have sought and found how to serve."
>
> —*Albert Schweitzer*

Before we can begin to give selflessly, our hearts must open to be able to recognize other people's needs. We then honor them by listening to what they need, and by providing what they ask rather than our opinion of it. As our hearts open further, we serve them without judgment, bathing them in compassion, allowing their dignity to be preserved. This kind of giving benefits both giver and receiver. In *Karma Yoga* we may perform the same duties and actions as before, but now our zeal is increased, just by letting go of expectations and results. For a little extra power, bring in the *Bhakti* (devotional) aspect and envision you are dedicating your actions to the Divine.

Every spiritual tradition encourages service as a way to purify the heart. To embark on our path of service, there are many reputable organizations you can participate in and support. In the beginning you may feel the desire to be recognized for your service: a thank-you letter, your name on a plaque, something of the sort. Giving anonymously can help limit this attachment. Also, at first you may feel more comfortable giving money than hands-on service. Slowly begin to give more of yourself and notice how it affects the rest of your life.

> "Letting go of attachment to the fruits of one's actions, one is ever content and does not have needs. Though one appears to be doing things (karma), actually the higher Self is the doer."
>
> —Bhagavad-Gita

We all carry impressions (*Samskaras*) from birth, early childhood, and even other lifetimes. The type of *Karma Yoga* you choose can help you to reduce the effects of any traumas and encourage healing. If you came from a poor family and are now financially comfortable, feeding people or donating clothing can make your heart sing. If you lost a parent at a young age, becoming a big sister to a young girl will be your joy. Customize *Karma Yoga* to your particular passion.

The Serenity Prayer seems to beautifully explain karma: "May I find the serenity to accept the things that cannot be changed, the courage to change the things that I can, and the wisdom to know the difference."

> "Never doubt that a small group of thoughtful, committed citizens can change the world. Indeed, it is the only thing that ever has."
>
> —Margaret Mead

The womb of karma (Karmasala), *sheathed by the* Kleshas *(veils), gives birth to experiences now and in the future.*

As long as the veils encase the womb of karma (Karmasala), *all actions will be affected.*

Karma bears fruits according to the type and quality of the seed planted, and the care given to its growth.

THE RIGHT LIVELIHOOD—DOES MONEY MOO?

"What about my work?" you may be thinking. "I need to earn a livelihood. I have a family to support! I cannot afford to donate *all my time!*"

"Choose a job you love and you will never have to work a day in your life."
—*Confucius*

Whatever service you perform in the world, let it be compatible with your spiritual path. If you sacrifice your inner convictions for the sake of money, you will always feel in debt, no matter what your bank balance may be. Even if your service in the world is not directly connected to your practice, unite it by serving all with a full heart.

The monetary compensation you receive carries the vibration of the work you do. For example, if you are a vegetarian for reasons of *ahimsa* (reverence for all life) and take a job selling meat in some way, you may find the lack of alignment unsettling. If out of necessity you *must* do that type of work, with each portion served, send a blessing to the animal's spirit. This will infuse the action with awareness and gratitude, allowing you to feel more at peace in your heart. If the contradiction continues to gnaw at you despite your best efforts, a change of profession may be necessary.

A poignant lesson was given to me during the time our ashram was building LOTUS (Light Of Truth Universal Shrine), an ecumenical shrine. As people would hear of the great endeavor to unite all religions under one holy roof, they would become inspired and want to donate. Some would come to give of their time; others would leave a monetary donation. After visiting for a few days, one very wealthy man resonated with what was taking place, and handed Sri Swamiji a check for a sizable donation. With a look of pleasant surprise, Sri Swamiji asked what the man did to earn such money. A bit shyly the man said, "Well, Swamiji, actually I am cattle rancher."

"So" said Swamiji, "you make your money raising cows and then sending them to the slaughterhouse?" The man replied that he did. Handing the man back his check, Swamiji told him, "You are always welcome to come and stay with us. But we cannot accept your money. It cries MOOO!"

Even something as subtle as what type of stock or bond you invest in affects you. If you keep your money in a bank and it earns interest, how is the bank investing that money? There are now socially responsible mutual funds that do not invest in weapons, alcohol, cigarettes, and so on. How you earn and invest your liveli-hood reverberates in everything it buys. Take time to know the company (*satsang*) your money is keeping. Earn it wisely.

When you perform an action, any action, offer *all results* to the highest good, and know that the deed will reverberate throughout your life. When you keep your heart in service, you can trust that all your needs will be cared for.

KARMA YOGA AND YOU

During these busy times, most of us consider it a luxury to take time to retreat from the world to the spirit, and it is touted as a blessing for the few. This is great *Karma Yoga* for us. When we feel nurtured, it is easy to nurture others. When we do not nurture our-selves, we are unable to draw upon qualities of love, faith, and other spiritual virtues. Not paying attention to our own needs causes them to burrow and hide deep within our hearts.

Karma Yoga for yourself can be even fifteen minutes to one hour a day. If you do it regularly, that short period of time is enough to revitalize body, mind, and emotions and lead you home to the spirit.

> "Always give from the overflow of your well, not from its depth."
>
> —*Sufi saying*

The good news is that Golden Age Consciousness is ripening right now. Many are acknowledging their spirituality and allowing it to blossom. With this rising group consciousness, the wheel of karma becomes a spiral that escalates us upward from the Iron Age to the Golden Age.

When the heart and spirit are held supreme, the Golden Age is now!

The womb of karma (Karmasala), *sheathed by the* Kleshas *(veils), gives birth to experiences now and in the future.*

As long as the veils encase the womb of karma (Karmasala), *all actions will be affected.*

Karma bears fruits according to the type and quality of the seed planted, and the care given to its growth.

EXPERIENCING A PAST KARMA THAT HAS A DIRECT EFFECT ON THE PRESENT

Remember a significant event in your life. You or someone else could have initiated it. Can you trace the experience of that occurrence and how it affected the next related incident? Do either of the original actions have reverberations even to the present?

It could be a teacher encouraging you to go on to college. Had she not handed you the college application along with papers for a scholarship, you might not have thought to apply for the monetary allotment. Because of her kindness, you were able to go to college and then law school, which allowed you years later to become a senator.

Go now the other way. Take an event in your life now and trace it back to when it was seeded. If the seed could be exchanged or replanted, how would it look different?

Next time you begin to do a significant action, think how the chain of events evolving from it will influence your life. You still have time to change it!

EXPERIENCING THE BLESSINGS OF *KARMA YOGA* (SELFLESS SERVICE) FOR OTHERS

Choose an aspect of service that you would like to offer. It could be for an individual or through an organization.

If at first you would like to donate money, that is a great start toward opening the heart. As time goes on, involve yourself more and more, finding a place to offer your goodwill that fits with your particular temperament.

Start to block off time regularly, on a weekly or monthly basis, for the service. Notice the excuses that come to keep you from doing it.

Convincing yourself to do the Seva (service), your heart begins to open. After a while you may find yourself canceling other events to enable you to do Karma Yoga! You soon begin to experience that the small amount you give is paled by the great joy you receive. Notice if the hurdles in your life become more relaxed.

EXPERIENCING THE BLESSINGS OF *KARMA YOGA* (SELFLESS SERVICE) FOR YOURSELF

In the midst of the busyness of life, find what feeds and nurtures you. In order for us to give lovingly to others, we need to feel the Divine within.

If your body is sore or aching, a luxurious bubble bath or a relaxing massage, even an extra couple of minutes in deep relaxation, can be profoundly healing. A sweet lay-down in the middle of the afternoon can feel like a week at the spa.

If it is the mind and emotions that pain you, remember to give them something fun to do, not always serious thoughts and feelings. Read a light and inspiring book, see a romantic comedy (that has nothing to do with your own relationship), do that art project you have been putting off, or just watch the simplicity of rain.

When you remember to serve yourself first, the service to others flows forth.

Make Karma Yoga *a steady habit. It encourages the wheel of karma, instead of spinning in a continuous circle, to spiral upward, taking you to the joy of your true nature.*

JNANA YOGA:
The Yoga of Intuitive Wisdom

HERE WE ARE introduced to the subtle power of Intuitive Wisdom, the grand wisdom of *Jnana Yoga*. These sutras are positioned at the seam of the physical and spiritual worlds. They perch us on the threshold of *Asthaangha Yoga* (the Eight-Faceted Path) where prudent insights are offered to sustain this pristine wisdom.

Intuitive Wisdom empowers us to expand beyond the constantly changing natural world (seen) to the abode of the Divine Spirit (seer).

With this understanding, once-vital difficulties become impotent.

The source of these difficulties is the inability to recognize the Divine Spirit (seer) as omniscient and therefore separate from the constantly changing natural world (seen).

When understood as illusory (Maya), nature (seen) and her attributes the gunas exist to serve the Divine Self (seer) with both enjoyment and liberation.

These attributes of nature (gunas) are both tangible and intangible.

The Divine Self (seer) observes the world without being affected by it.

The natural world (seen) exists for benefit of the Divine Self (seer).

With realization of the Divine Self (seer), the illusory natural world (seen) becomes transparent, though still seemingly very real to those enmeshed in it.

When the Divine Self (seer) and nature (seen) unite, this dynamic and powerful synergy creates the illusory world, obscuring the vision of spirit.

This union is consummated when we forget the Divine Self (seer).

With constant remembrance of the Divine Self, no such union is possible.

Established in the grace of Intuitive Wisdom, we experience liberation.

Liberation is recognized in seven ways: when we no longer feel the need for knowledge, to stay away from anything or anyone, to gather material things, or to act. Our constant companions are joy, faith, and clarity.

II.15 *Intuitive Wisdom empowers us to expand beyond the constantly changing natural world (seen) to the abode of the Divine Spirit (seer).*

As our consciousness expands, we realize that there is an essential difference between the inner world of the spirit and the outer world of nature. An Intuitive Wisdom emerges, strengthened by constant acknowledgment. Our intuition whispers to us in a voice that is often overshadowed by the louder, more prominent voice of our thoughts. It is the quiet voice of our Spirit guiding us toward the light. That Intuitive Wisdom is always to be trusted, as it springs from the gratitude of knowing. It cannot be influenced by messages of this changing world; rather, it is rooted in unchanging reality.

Elisabeth Kübler-Ross, a noble pioneer in the field of end-of-life care, was often asked if she believed in reincarnation. Her quick-witted reply was "I do not believe in reincarnation—I know it to be true!"

As our intuition develops, the perception that our life is formed from outside influences is welcomingly transformed, and we gain the knowledge that the True Self is the primary influence. All tangible world experiences are delivered by our senses and interpreted by our thoughts and emotions. That which is material is temporary and causes us to regret its passing. We understand that the world does not have the capacity to secure our everlasting happiness. The more we understand the complexity of nature's effect on us, the more effortlessly we are able to expand beyond her grasp and align with our true knowledge.

> "When we are able to know the Self, all else is known."
> —*Bhagavad-Gita*

WISDOM FROM THE HEART

Most often *Jnana Yoga* is described from a purely mental perspective using terms like "reason," "discernment," and "discrimination." These words are fitting if we are addressing wisdom only from the mental perspective. Wisdom also comes from the heart, as intuition.

Directing our lives from our Intuitive Wisdom, nothing is deemed good or bad. We are simply able to observe where the tossing *gunas* have temporarily lighted. We may find we are happy to see a friend one minute, unhappy to see her the next. All this has to do with the way the mind and emotions are playing out at that very moment. The effects of past conditions can cause strong reactions if we are not vigilant. *Patterns are difficult to change.* As we recognize the True Self, everything else in the world becomes secondary. Any desire to possess or run from the world is dissipated. Instead in our stillness it comes to us.

When you understand the physical world, there is nothing to hinder you from playing and having fun with everything. At first it may seem overwhelming to experience the world in this unusual way, but like any other skill you learn, the ease and joy come as you become more proficient.

When you were young, were you afraid to ride a bike? "How could I possibly balance on those thin tires? How do I steer, and more importantly how do I stop?" In the beginning you had to use training wheels while someone vigilantly held onto your bicycle's seat. After a while the training wheels were removed, but that attentive protector still held firm to your seat, until finally one day, although you were shaky, you rode alone. That was many years ago and not even a whisper of doubt joins you as you now mount your bike. Only the freedom and joy remain, making the whole world your playground.

The real power comes when we can expand beyond the constant changes in nature and be firmly grounded in our Intuitive Wisdom.

Intuitive Wisdom empowers us to expand beyond the constantly changing natural world (seen) to the abode of the Divine Spirit (seer).

11.16 *With this understanding, once-vital difficulties become impotent.*

11.17 *The source of these difficulties is the inability to recognize the Divine Spirit (seer) as omniscient and therefore separate from the constantly changing natural world (seen).*

11.18 *When understood as illusory* (Maya), *nature (seen) and her attributes the* gunas *exist to serve the Divine Self (seer) with both enjoyment and liberation.*

Here Yoga Wisdom introduces us to two distinct aspects: the one who *sees* (the True Self) and that which is *seen* (everything else). Most of the time we identify with what is *seen* rather than with the one who sees. Difficulties manifest because we do not understand that everything in this natural world changes and cannot be slowed, halted, or possessed. The *only thing we can hold onto* is the knowledge of the True Self.

Once upon a time there was a great queen. Graced by realizing the eternal truth that ultimately she could not possess anything, she decided to free all her possessions. She issued a proclamation to the entire principality, offering her worldly goods to anyone who wanted them. The only restriction was that the treasures could not leave the palace until after the stroke of five o'clock on the appointed day.

It was four fifty-five on the day of this great giveaway and all were eagerly standing by their selected prizes. A strange and imposing woman entered the palace. The queen greeted her and immediately apologized because everything of value had already been claimed. This did not faze the woman in the least; just before the stroke of five, she took her place next to the queen and inquired calmly, "Your Majesty, when you said *everything* in the palace was to be given away, did that also include *you?*"

Surprised and bewildered, the queen stammered, "I did say *everything;* I guess that means me too." Then, the woman said boldly, "I choose *you!*" "But why," stammered the queen, "would you want *me?* I am now penniless." Embracing the queen at the exact stroke of five, the woman proclaimed, "Everyone *stop* where you are! No one is to leave the palace until all the treasures are returned to their rightful places." Laughing, she continued to enlighten the people, "You went for the small trinkets, but *I* have chosen the greatest treasure of all, the queen. Because when I possess *her,* I possess *everything!*"

It is not only the material possessions that we want to hold onto, but also the desire for our bodies and minds to either stay the same or be different from what they are. When we are young, we want to look and act grown up. When we are graying, we add color so we can look younger. Once we realize that everything in nature changes, we liberate ourselves from wanting things to be different than they actually are. We enjoy every moment.

An interesting way to observe this phenomenon is to browse through a photo album that captures you from childhood up to the present day. Start at the beginning and try to remember how you felt and thought at that moment in time. You may not remember as far back as infancy, but notice at what age the memories start. Then progressively go through the photos noting how you felt at those frozen moments in your story. Observe the snapshots of yourself on your first day at school or at a ballet lesson. Even though the body size is smaller and your wants and needs may differ, isn't there something deep inside you that feels the same? Can you detect a similar awareness weaving through your entire life? There is an interior sameness, which never changes, a presence watching, guiding us; it is our *Intuitive Wisdom*.

I remember my mother at age ninety-one emphatically calling me to her room. "Look," she said, gesturing to the mirror. I looked but was unable to discern what the surprising discovery was. "There." She pointed. "Who is that old woman looking back at me? It can't be me. I'm not that old, am I?"

It does seem to happen so fast. One day we are playing grown-up wearing our mother's high heels, then at what seems like the next moment, *our children* are playing grown-up with *our things*. That is the temperament of the changing world: the only constancy is within.

If we trust our Intuitive Wisdom, everything can be enjoyable because we have found the magic wand to convert everything that life brings into joy.

With this understanding, once-vital difficulties become impotent.

The source of these difficulties is the inability to recognize the Divine Spirit (seer) as omniscient and therefore separate from the constantly changing natural world (seen).

When understood as illusory (Maya), nature (seen) and her attributes the gunas exist to serve the Divine Self (seer) with both enjoyment and liberation.

II.19 *These attributes of nature* (gunas) *are both tangible and intangible.*

There are various stages to the manifestation of the *gunas*. Some are apparent as our senses inform us how things are now and how they then change. We are less aware of the intangible changes. Most of us have not developed the resources to grasp that which we are unable to know with the senses. As we develop our inner perception, we are able to know that we know what there is to know.

When nature began it was indefinite and without expression. From this stage the *gunas* (attributes of nature) formed and were in balance. As the universe evolved, the *gunas* began to shift dominance, and the world as we know it came into being. The *buddhi* (intellect), *ahamkara* (thoughts and emotions), and *manas* (senses) that we spoke about earlier manifested from the disproportionate interplay of the *gunas*.

In a way it is like baking bread. First, we have the idea of bread and how it will taste and how to make it. The next is actually gathering the ingredients, which vary in quantity according to the type of bread we are baking. Then we mix the individual measured ingredients together until they form dough ready to be kneaded. Sometimes we must add more flour or water to make the consistency just right. It then is allowed to rise, before being baked in the oven. It is only when it is in its totally manifested state (baked and cooled) that we employ our senses to eat and enjoy it.

These attributes of nature (gunas) *are both tangible and intangible.*

11.20 *The Divine Self (seer) observes the world without being affected by it.*

11.21 *The natural world (seen) exists for benefit of the Divine Self (seer).*

11.22 *With realization of the Divine Self (seer), the illusory natural world (seen) becomes transparent, though still seemingly very real to those enmeshed in it.*

11.23 *When the Divine Self (seer) and nature (seen) unite, this dynamic and powerful synergy creates the illusory world, obscuring the vision of spirit.*

11.24 *This union is consummated when we forget the Divine Self (seer).*

11.25 *With constant remembrance of the Divine Self, no such union is possible.*

At this point you may be wondering, "If life *could be simpler* if we kept our awareness on the Divine Self, why are we not designed to do that?" We *are designed* to make the decision where to direct our awareness. But most of us choose to keep it focused on the material world, perpetuating the *grand illusion (Maha Maya)* of life. However, it is only an illusion to those who understand that it is an illusion. To the rest, it seems *very real*.

AWAKING FROM THE DREAM

Illusion (*Maya*) in this sense is like a waking dream. While we are dreaming (either during the day or night), it *appears* to be very real. Measuring a person's physiological responses during an active dream state reveals that the blood pressure rises along with the heart rate. The eyes dart back and forth; sometimes the legs and arms move as if running. If you sleep with another person, you may have even gotten *kicked or poked* during one of his very active dreams.

Most of the time when we awaken, we quickly become aware that we had been dreaming. Other times, though, we are *unable* to differentiate the dream state from the waking state. If it is a wonderful dream, we do not want to let go of it; in other cases, as much as we want to awaken from it, an unhappy dream creeps into our waking state. This is the way of *Maya*. Unless we are able to completely wake up our consciousness, we constantly dwell in a waking dream. When we do experience enlightenment, we wake up and realize it was all an illusion, unreal.

This morning you may have looked outside and said, "I do not want to go for a walk today; the sun is not shining." At midnight you might doubt the existence of the sun since it is nowhere to be seen. In our minds we all know that the sun is always there, even though sometimes it is engulfed by clouds or on the other side of the earth from us. Even when the sun is hidden, it remains the life-giving force that sustains our physical existence. In the same way, our True Self transmits life force to the body, mind, and emotions, but because we cannot *see* the True Self or *experience* it as real, we doubt its existence.

PLAYING THE FOOL

Mula Nasrudin was a great Sufi mystic whose method of teaching was to play the part of the fool. (He *purposely* played that part!) One fine day one of his disciples questioned him, "Oh, great Mula, which is more important: the sun or the moon?"

He answered without hesitation. "The moon, of course. During the day the sun is not so important because there is already light. But at night the moon is vital because it is our only source of light." He tried to trick them into thinking that the moon is self-effulgent like the sun, not merely the reflection of the sun's rays. Can we trick ourselves into remembering that our thoughts, emotions, and intellect are not self-effulgent but merely a reflection? They are reflections that come from either the external material world or the light within. Often it is difficult to discern their origin.

Much of the time our identity is molded by who *we think we are* and by the feedback we receive from others, rather than from the eternal light. As we cultivate our Intuitive Wisdom, the light of the Self clearly and brightly influences all dimensions of us. In this elevated consciousness, when you are unhappy, *you know* you are unhappy; when you are happy, *you know* you are happy. You then become the knower in all conditions. And nature is here to help us become liberated.

The Divine Self (seer) observes the world without being affected by it.

The natural world (seen) exists for benefit of the Divine Self (seer).

With realization of the Divine Self (seer), the illusory natural world (seen) becomes transparent, though still seemingly very real to those enmeshed in it.

When the Divine Self (seer) and nature (seen) unite, this dynamic and powerful synergy creates the illusory world, obscuring the vision of spirit.

This union is consummated when we forget the Divine Self (seer).

With constant remembrance of the Divine Self, no such union is possible.

11.26 *Established in the grace of Intuitive Wisdom, we experience liberation.*

This is the key to freedom. By constant observation through Intuitive Wisdom, we know that we are the eternal unchanging Self. If spirit (seer) and nature (seen) give us opposite experiences, we are able to recognize the Self (seer) only through the depth of our Intuitive Wisdom and knowledge. When they unite for the purpose of freedom, nature (seen) helps us to find and reflect the eternal Self (seer).

Whatever you think, so you become. If you believe you are limited, you will be limited; if you believe you are free, you are free.

There is a wonderful strategy that is used to train an elephant to stay in one place. At an early age, the elephant has a large, thick chain attached to her foot. If she tries to stray, the strong chain gives the signal to go no farther. As the baby elephant grows in strength, a large rope replaces the heavy chain. The tether continues to *decrease* in size and strength until the elephant is fully grown.

This may seem counterintuitive, but it is not possible to find a chain or rope strong enough to restrain the huge adult animal. With this training, though, a small cord does the job. Because her memory holds the experience of being restricted by a chain stronger than her baby muscles could resist, the grown elephant assumes that the small cord continues to bind her.

How many tethers are still holding us attached to our minds and emotions?

Through constant observation the distinction between the changing qualities of what is perceived and the unchanging quality of what perceives becomes evident.

"The (one) who has no inner life is the slave of (her/his) surroundings."
—Henri Frederic Amiel

Established in the grace of Intuitive Wisdom, we experience liberation.

II.27 *Liberation is recognized in seven ways: we no longer feel the need for knowledge, to stay away from anything or anyone, to gather material things, or to act. Our constant companions are joy, faith, and clarity.*

There are different ways to interpret the various wisdom paths to freedom. Some view it as gradual, as if experiencing the dawn, where each moment the magnitude of the light becomes greater and greater, until it is seen in its totality. With this view our longing for material things and even our thirst for knowledge dwindles in the promising presence of the eternal. Along with the light there is an ever-quickening dawning of joy, faith, and clarity. (This is considered the *Bhakti* [devotional] way to enlightenment.)

The other way is not gradual; rather, it suggests that after all the practices have aligned, consciousness spontaneously illuminates. This view is more reminiscent of turning on a light switch than of a gradual dawning. It holds the same yearnings, and through will-power it encourages the casting away of material effects that impede the way. (This is considered the *Jnani* way to enlightenment.)

While there are many who tout *Jnana Yoga* as a direct and expedient way to merge with eternal light, it seems to be a matter of temperament. Both are tried-and-true paths to the Divine. Embrace whatever avenue you feel most in tune with; there are always benefits to balance in both.

A *JNANI*, A *BHAKTI,* AND A PILE OF PEANUTS

Observe two people eating peanuts. Can you distinguish the *Jnani* (student of Intuitive Wisdom) from the *Bhakti* (devotee)? The first one cracks the shell and immediately pops the sweet kernel into her mouth, delighting in the taste before going on to the next nut. The other person unshells the nut and carefully places it in a pile, savoring the delicacy for the time when all the nuts are ready.

The first person has the personality more fitting a *Bhakti* because she wants to taste the sweetness all the way through the process. The second person, not wanting to be distracted from her mission, looks forward to eating the whole pile after accomplishing the unsheathing and sorting. The *Bhakti* is similar to the dawning light and the *Jnani* is more like the light switch. The end result is the same: they remember they are one with the Divine Self.

"Beholding the Self by the Self, one is satisfied in the Self."
—*Bhagavad-Gita*

Having written all this about *Jnana Yoga,* I urge you to resist the temptation to get *too* caught up in esoteric philosophy. While it is important to know why we are doing the practices, it can also be a way of corralling us toward intellectual gymnastics, leaving the True Self still occluded. *Philosophy without practice is ineffective; practice without philosophy is precarious. Asthaanga Yoga,* the eight-faceted path that follows, offers practices that bring the *Jnana Yoga* sutras into our daily life.

Liberation is recognized in seven ways: we no longer feel the need for knowledge, to stay away from anything or anyone, to gather material things, or to act. Our constant companions are joy, faith, and clarity.

EXPERIENCING WHO YOU ARE BY KNOWING WHAT YOU ARE NOT

Have the body in a comfortable position, spine erect, shoulders relaxed. Begin to observe the body. Check to see if everything is relaxed—your toes, feet, ankles, shins, calves, knees, thighs, hips, hands, wrists, forearms, etc.

Inhale through the nose. As you exhale through the nose, let your breath out very slowly—and with it, relax. Take in another breath and let it out even more slowly. Feel yourself relaxing deeply.

Place the awareness of I in the center of the heart.
Ask yourself: Who am I?
Am I the body? The flesh? The bones? The blood? The organs?
No, I am not the body!
Who am I?
Am I the organs of motion?
Am I the arms that reach out? No, I am not the arms or the action of reaching.
Who am I?
Am I the legs that propel the body to move and touch the earth?
No, I am not the legs or the movement of the legs.
Who am I?
Am I the organs of the senses?

Am I the eyes that see all sights? No, I am not the eyes or the seeing!

Who am I?

Am I the ears that hear all sounds? No, I am not the ears or the hearing.

Who am I?

Am I the nose that smells all scents? No, I am not the nose or the smelling.

Who am I?

Am I the tongue that tastes and talks? No, I am not the tongue or the sense of taste or the action of speech.

Who am I?

Am I the skin, the sense of feeling? No, I am not the skin or the sense of touch.

Who am I?

Observe and experience the following:

your eyes and inner and outer seeing

your ears and inner and outer hearing

your nose and inner and outer smells

your tongue and inner and outer tasting

your tongue and inner and outer talking

Who am I?

Am I the mind?

No, I am not the mind.

How could I be the mind if I am observing the mind? I must be something other than the mind.

Who am I?

Am I the emotions?

No, I am not the emotions because I can observe and change the emotions.

Who am I?

Even the original I that was put in the center of the heart is not me. Because I put it there.

Who am I?
I am beyond all these things. I am Absolute Truth, Absolute
Knowledge, Absolute Bliss.
Who am I?
I am the one who knows.

ASTHAANGA YOGA:
The Eight-Faceted Path

WE FIND THE practical application of Yogic Wisdom distilled into eight dynamic facets. As you were studying the preceding sutras, you might have wondered, "How can *I* possibly realize this?" The answer lies in *Asthaanga Yoga*. It is so often considered the essence that, for many, the whole study of the sutras is termed *Asthaanga Yoga*.

By embracing **Asthaanga Yoga,** *the Eight-Faceted Path, Intuitive Wisdom dawns and reveals our inner radiance.*

Asthaanga Yoga, *the Eight-Faceted Path, embraces:*
Yama: *reflection of our true nature*
Niyama: *evolution toward harmony*
Asana: *comfort in being, posture*
Pranayama: *enhancement and guidance of*
universal prana *(energy)*
Pratyahara: *encouraging the senses to draw within*
Dharana: *gathering and focusing of consciousness inward*
Dhyana: *continuous inward flow of consciousness*
Samadhi: *union with Divine Consciousness.*

Yama *(reflection of our true nature) is experienced through:*
Ahimsa: *reverence, love, compassion for all*
Satya: *truthfulness, integrity*

Astheya: *generosity, honesty*
Brahmacharya: *balance and moderation*
of the vital life force
Aparigraha: *awareness of abundance, fulfillment.*

These great truths are universal and inherent to all beings.
If altered or ignored, the quality of life is greatly compromised.

Niyama (*evolution toward harmony*) *encompasses:*
Saucha: *simplicity, purity, refinement*
Santosha: *contentment, being at peace with*
oneself and others
Tapas: *igniting the purifying flame*
Swadhaya: *sacred study of the Divine through scripture,*
nature, and introspection
Iswara Pranidhana: *wholehearted dedication to the Divine.*

When presented with disquieting thoughts or feelings, cultivate
an opposite, elevated attitude. This is Pratipaksha Bhavana.

The desire to act upon unwholesome thoughts or actions or to
cause or condone others toward these thoughts or actions is
preventable. This is also Pratipaksha Bhavana.

11.28 *By embracing* Asthaanga Yoga, *the Eight-Faceted Path, Intuitive Wisdom dawns and reveals our inner radiance.*

11.29 Asthaanga Yoga, *the Eight-Faceted Path,* embraces:

> *Yama:* reflection of our true nature
> *Niyama:* evolution toward harmony
> *Asana:* comfort in being, posture
> *Pranayama:* enhancement and guidance of universal prana (energy)
> *Pratyahara:* encouraging the senses to draw within
> *Dharana:* gathering and focusing of consciousness inward
> *Dhyana:* continuous inward flow of consciousness
> *Samadhi:* union with Divine Consciousness.

Asthaanga is two words. *Astha* means "eight" and *angha* means "intertwining facets." *Angha* is often translated as "limb," and the term can give the impression of a linear ascent, like climbing a tree. Starting at the trunk we wend our way out to the end of the limb. But instead of a completion, the limbs of this tree end in interconnection. This may be frustrating when we are unable to complete each one in its own turn. But it is an integrated system.

Rather than the image of a single tree or limb, the many facets of *Asthaanga Yoga* are similar to a grove of trees. From the trunk upward, the trees appear to be independent, not connected to one another. However, if we venture several inches below the surface, we will find that these seemingly separate trees have their root systems intertwined. Their interdependency on one another for enduring strength and drawing in moisture unites them. Each is able to manifest a unique appearance while embracing the same consciousness. Similar to entwined tree roots, we are reminded that *Asthaanga* is not a series of practices to "accomplish"; rather, it is an offering of infinite possibilities and combinations to enhance our way of being. Because of this we encourage them to interact and function interdependently rather than individually. At times we may choose to single out one or another to help us focus on a particular aspect of our development. After some time, the integration of the other facets will be necessary as we continue our journey inward toward wholeness and discovering our divinity.

Five of these facets are described in the second book, "*Sadhana Pada*: Cultivation of Spiritual Practice." The last three are expounded upon in the third book, "*Vibhuti Pada*: The Divine Manifestation of Power." This structure is meant to suggest that *Dharana* (contemplation), *Dhyana* (meditation), and *Samadhi* (Union with Divine Consciousness) are not practices in themselves, but states that blossom through the nurturing practices that preceded them.

Through the process of incarnation, our finite bodies must accommodate the vast and infinite ocean of consciousness, as it infuses Divine qualities into our human life. As human beings, we hope to reflect the higher states of consciousness along with our humanity. The Eight-Faceted Path encourages that integration.

Asthaanga Yoga *is the Eight-Faceted Path.*

11.30 Yama *(reflection of our true nature) is experienced through:*

>   *Ahimsa:* reverence, love, compassion for all
>   *Satya:* truthfulness, integrity
>   *Astheya:* generosity, honesty
>   *Brahmacharya:* balance and moderation
>   of the vital life force
>   *Aparigraha:* awareness of abundance,
>   fulfillment.

THE TWO PINNACLES OF DYNAMIC ENERGY

Yama (reflection of our true nature) and *Niyama* (evolution toward harmony) are the first two facets of *Asthaanga.*

Within the two facets, *Yama* and *Niyama,* there are five additional facets encouraging us to live in peace, honoring the spirit at each moment. Imagine two round brilliant cut diamonds meshed together at the top, each directing energy to or from the pinnacle. The pinnacles represent the foremost qualities of each: *Ahimsa* in *Yama* and *Iswara Pranidhana* in *Niyama.* When we revere all as ourselves through *Ahimsa,* the other four qualities of *Yama: Satya,* (truthfulness), *Astheya* (generosity), *Brahmacharya* (moderation), and *Aparigraha* (abundance) are naturally present.

Iswara Pranidhana, wholehearted dedication to the Divine, conveys the essence of the four other *Niyamas: Saucha* (simplicity), *Santosha* (contentment), *Tapas* (igniting the purifying flame), and *Swadhaya* (sacred study). The integration of the *Yamas* and *Niyamas* in our lives reflects the beauty and light of a diamond. Everything that is touched by these will then reproduce its own beauty and light.

INSPIRED OFFERINGS, NOT COMMANDMENTS

Often, to simplify the enormous breadth and depth of the *Yamas* and *Niyamas,* they are called the "Do's and Don'ts of Yoga" or sometimes the "Ten Commandments of Yoga." This is taking a highly refined and virtuous way of living expressed throughout the millennia and reducing it to a finger-shaking image: "If you do not do this or that, you will be punished." When observed on a subtler level, the *Yamas* and *Niyamas* seem to be more of a tribute to being, affirming our already Divine nature.

During the time period when the Ten Commandments were delivered, the Divine was represented as a strong and very strict patriarch. The people's morals and attitudes had diminished and many thought that drastic measures were needed to facilitate a change.

During the time when the ideals of the *Yamas* and *Niyamas* were formulated, the atmosphere was of a different nature. It was during the Golden Age *(Sat Yuga),* and virtue still reigned. Nonetheless, the steady decline in consciousness was evident. Everyone was eager to find a way to preserve these values. The positive way people lived their lives was reflected in their wisdom.

Yama: *reflection of our true nature.*

It is up to each of us in our hearts to decide which level of consciousness we want to abide in, in our spiritual life and in the world. As you read and practice the *Yamas* and *Niyamas,* feel that they are sparking your Golden Age *(Sat Yuga)* consciousness where virtue is supreme. These two giant pyramids of virtue are given to us so that we may remember to live our lives in a noble and sacred way.

Knowing the importance of repeating a statement in the affirmative, I have chosen to translate (as much as I possibly could) using positive, life-affirming language. If we say, "I will *not* eat sugar today," the human mind sees through the "not" and concentrates on the sugar. In the same way, continually reading translations formed in the negative evokes Iron Age *(Kali Yuga)* consciousness, rather than our natural effulgence shining through from the Golden Age *(Sat Yuga).*

When an athlete is in training, positive phrasing is found to be most effective. "Don't put your elbows out when you swing that golf club" may actually cause the undesirable effect. Instead, "Keep your elbows in when you swing" is found to elicit better results.

When words or phrases evoke fear, punishment, or denial of pleasure, they encroach on our spiritual practices and diminish rather than enhance the glory of our true nature. By embracing everything as Divine, our all-loving nature is radiantly revealed.

Bring forth the Golden Age *(Sat Yuga)* consciousness within the Iron Age *(Kali Yuga)* by upholding these Divine qualities. Be open-hearted as the facets of *Asthaanga Yoga* unfurl the realization of your true nature.

Yama: *reflection of our true nature.*

II.3I *These great truths are universal and inherent to all beings. If altered or ignored, the quality of life is greatly compromised.*

We can all make excuses and find reasons for not upholding these declarations, even when our quality of life is affected. The infractions may seem so *minor* that they remain unnoticed; yet, some part of us is deeply affected. In those quiet moments by ourselves, we find the incongruities between who we are and who we think we are emerging. They tend to be so subtle that although we may be aware that something is bothering us, we are unable to discern its origin. If something is said that inadvertently awakens those opposing thoughts and feelings, we may overreact without understanding the real cause of the distress.

One of the most important ways to keep our intention is the power of *satsang* (company of those who share the same truth). When we need reassurance to stay focused on the practices, who do we call on? If it is someone who already has experienced the benefits of practice, we will receive encouragement to continue. Without the same understanding, a well-meaning friend might convince us to venture onward to other horizons.

The Yama and Niyama are expressed in all aspects of our thoughts, words, and actions. This is what allows them to be at the same time powerful and challenging to abide by.

These great truths are universal and inherent to all beings. If altered or ignored, the quality of life is greatly compromised.

II.32 Niyama *(evolution toward harmony)* encompasses:

Saucha: simplicity, purity, refinement

Santosha: contentment, being at peace with oneself and others

Tapas: igniting the purifying flame

Swadhaya: sacred study of the Divine through scripture, nature, and introspection

Iswara Pranidhana: wholehearted dedication to the Divine.

Here *Iswara Pranidhana* is at the pinnacle of the diamond pyramid. All of the *Niyamas* are enhanced when *Iswara Pranidhana* is honored, and it is honored when we live in harmony with the other four *Niyamas*.

Niyama: *evolution toward harmony.*

11.33 *When presented with disquieting thoughts or feelings, cultivate an opposite, elevated attitude. This is* Pratipaksha Bhavana.

This is one of my favorite sutras because it helps to change *my* attitude rather than hoping to change the situation or the people who "cause me" to be unhappy. It is a key practice that enables us to remain in harmony, balanced, and openhearted.

Pratipaksha offers the option of cultivating the opposite thoughts, feelings, and actions. *Bhavana* is the Sanskrit root of our English verb "to be." Together they encourage us to reverse our attitude, to embrace a noble way of being.

Daily life presents us with a plethora of frustrations and challenges. Our hope is that as our consciousness blossoms, life's trials will ease. It is not always the case; often the situations that were previously endured gracefully affect us *more*. With clarity we realize that changing the situation may not be possible; rather we see that changing our attitude allows peace to bloom.

We may stubbornly hold the belief that others cause our problems and inconveniences. In those situations we may appoint ourselves as their teachers to show them the correct way to act. From that attitude our egos enlarge, leaving us with less room for insight. If you routinely feel it is the other person's fault, take another look, this time from a different perspective.

When presented with disquieting thoughts or feelings, cultivate an opposite, elevated attitude. This is Pratipaksha Bhavana.

Pratipaksha Bhavana is a simple and direct way of keeping our minds calm and our hearts open. How often during the day do unwanted thoughts or feelings pop up to disturb your calm? Some days there might be too many to count!

When we are aware of these unfavorable attitudes *before* they manifest as word or action, we retain the power to reverse them. Do you feel fear? Cultivate courage. Anger? Cultivate love. Try substituting not just a word but a whole scene or action. Perhaps you are in the midst of a heated discussion with your spouse, when from another room you hear your sweet baby cooing. Chances are as soon as you hear the first sound, your mind and heart will leave the disagreement, and your anger will melt away as your heart opens to your child. The next time you feel annoyed with anyone, invoke an image like the face of your sweet baby, or perhaps a budding flower or a brilliant sunset. The person worthy of your discontent may suddenly appear more vulnerable as you feel more loving. The best part is that you both reap the benefits.

MAKE A DIFFICULT PERSON YOUR PERSONAL DEITY

There was a time while living at the ashram that I was in charge of a large department with many ashramites to supervise. One quite grumpy monk very much resented doing anything that was asked of him, especially if a woman issued the directive. Each morning, I dreaded telling him the needs of the day. He remained quiet as he stood in front of me, but as he turned and walked away he would mutter unkind words. It very much disturbed me, but no amount of words or gestures could soothe him.

Calling on *Pratipaksha Bhavana,* I designed a spiritual practice in which he was the principal deity. Each day as he entered my office, I would imagine placing a garland of flowers over his head and touching his feet. As he turned to walk·away, murmuring under his breath, my hands joined together in a *pranam* to wish him well.

This "worship" continued and initiated itself each time he passed by. The practice then sprung into being each time I thought about him. Of course, no one else knew about it; only my mind and heart held the secret.

One week into the practice, I was no longer stifling a visceral reaction to run when I saw him. The practice was benefiting me in many ways. My mind and heart were now focusing on flower garlands and worship, rather than dwelling on a strategy to avoid grumpy people.

One morning, at the usual time, he appeared in my office and, with a surprised tone, said, "You know that I do not like you very much, don't you?" I only nodded my head "yes," so as to not give my voice a chance to betray me. "Well, it's a funny thing," he continued, "but in the last week, I find that I am actually starting to look forward to seeing you, well, just a little bit. I can't figure out why. Do you know?"

Smiling on the inside, I said, "Well, perhaps we are both changing and our reason for disliking each other is fading away." I kept up the practice for months. I cannot say we became best friends, but we both were able to say, "We like each other."

When presented with disquieting thoughts or feelings, cultivate an opposite, elevated attitude. This is **Pratipaksha Bhavana.**

EXPERIENCING THE PROFOUND EFFECT
OF CHANGING YOUR ATTITUDE

Sit comfortably.

Think of a quality that you would like to invite into your life. A simple one- or two-word phrase is best. It could be "peace," "joy," "cooperation," "adaptability," etc. (For this example we will use "joy".)

Bring forth an aspect of yourself that no longer fosters the person you want to be. Can you tell where in your body it is stored? If possible, put a name to it—"self-righteousness," "stubbornness," "anger," etc. (For this example we will use "resentment.")

Now, choose a quality that you would like to send out to the world. It could be the same or a different one than you chose to bring into your life. (For this example we will use the quality of "peace".)

Begin to take in and release deep, full breaths.

As you breathe in, allow the mind and heart to integrate the quality of joy into your being. Feel joy infusing each cell, encircling the place where you are holding resentment, and allow the unwanted feeling to dissipate.

As you breathe out, let joy transform resentment into peace and send it as your wish for the world.

(When the mind is focused as in this practice, it is important not to hold the breath or breathe out the negative emotion. Through the breath the mind gains power, and with focus the negative is exaggerated, rather than calmed. It is fun to watch the resentment dissolve and transform into peace!)

EXPERIENCING THE EFFECTS THIS HAS ON DIFFICULT PEOPLE AND SITUATIONS

As you feel comfortable with the previous practice, use it in a variety of situations with people or things that cause you to become annoyed.

Begin to breathe in a positive quality (it could be the same or different than you used in the last practice); as you breathe out, send a directed wish to them.

To add to the power, notice something you like about that person. That alone is enough to change your vibrational quality. (The thing you like about the person might be as simple as a pretty blouse or the color of a necktie.)

Continue the imagery until the negative feelings subside or you are able to remove yourself from the circumstances. If it is a situation you frequently encounter, repeat this practice as often as possible and be amazed at the change in both you and them.

II.34 *The desire to act upon unwholesome thoughts or actions or to cause or condone others toward these thoughts or actions is preventable. This is also* Pratipaksha Bhavana.

Even the *desire* to do something hurtful to another can be pacified by *Pratipaksha Bhavana*. This also encompasses the impulse to stand by and allow hurtful actions to happen to others. There are situations in which we may feel helpless given the actions being taken either by an individual or a government. Sometimes our only recourse is to peacefully protest, petition, write letters, or speak out in some way. Through this we may assuage our exasperation and hope that our intervention will elicit some benefit.

It seems like many years ago that I discovered that the simple act of eating a grape was contributing to the suffering of many. Learning the grape pickers' plight, many of us joined together in a boycott, our hearts leaping in solidarity. Even now, a long time hence, this self-imposed act of camaraderie makes me hesitate when popping a tasty grape in my mouth.

We hear much about companies using child labor or abusing workers. Taking action even in the smallest way (such as not buying the product) allows the mind and the heart to know they are contributing to the solution, not the problem.

It is important for retaining our peace that the protests, boycotts, letters, and petitions are arranged in a calm nature. Otherwise, we unknowingly contribute to the injury. When participating in a peace demonstration, remember to bring your peace with you and keep it strong. It is from this cocoon of peace that the power emerges.

The desire to act upon unwholesome thoughts or actions or to cause or condone others toward these thoughts or actions is preventable. This is also Pratipaksha Bhavana.

YAMA:
Reflection of Our True Nature

HERE WE EXPLORE FIVE inner facets of *Asthaanga Yoga* called *Yama*. They encourage us to live in peace with ourselves and one another.

Embracing reverence and love for all (Ahimsa), we experience oneness.

Dedicated to truth and integrity (Satya), our thoughts, words, and actions gain the power to manifest.

Abiding in generosity and honesty (Astheya), material and spiritual prosperity is bestowed.

Devoted to living a balanced and moderate life (Brahmacharya), the scope of one's life force becomes boundless.

Acknowledging abundance (Aparigraha), we recognize the blessings in everything and gain insights into the purpose of our worldly existence.

11.35 *Embracing reverence and love for all* (Ahimsa), *we experience oneness.*

Ahimsa, the pinnacle of the diamond pyramid, gives brilliance to the *Yamas.* Sanctifying every moment of the day with reverence and love, the other four *Yamas* easily integrate into our lives.

The practice of *Ahimsa* transports us to Golden Age (*Sat Yuga*) awareness, where the entire world of people, animals, plants, and inanimate objects is our family and friends, and ultimately we are one.

> "To those that lowly creep, I am the self in all."
>
> —*Swami Vivekananda*

As babies, we see the world through pure hearts and open eyes. We live the purity of *Ahimsa,* experiencing oneness with everyone and everything. With the development of the mind's ability to discriminate, differences emerge. We must then be constantly reminded that even though people and things appear to be different, in our essence we are all the same.

Throughout time, many religious stories and books underplayed the loving and compassionate aspect of the Divine, accentuating instead the fearful and punitive roles. Fear, rationalized the storytellers, would have the power to make us humble and thus believe in virtuous rules.

THE MASCULINE AND FEMININE QUALITIES IN THE SACRED TEXTS

The (masculine) qualities of fury and punishment in the Old and New Testaments cry out for balance. Clandestinely woven throughout the Hebrew Bible is the term *rachamim,* the feminine quality of mercy and compassion that is attributed to God's softer side. Its meaning is derived from *rechem,* meaning maternal or womblike attributes. *Rachamim* perpetuates the dynamic regenerative power millions have felt from this great scripture for thousands of years. With the translation into modern languages, the representation and wording of the feminine are obscured, and the masculine qualities are brought front and center. It is important to remember that all life is a balance, and a delicate one at that.

The New Testament has the benefit of the great parables of Jesus' compassion. Throughout the scripture, he is constantly coming to the defense of the wrongly accused and the outcasts of society, showing us that we are all the same in our hearts. Depending upon who is narrating, the compassion is underscored or overlooked. The appearances and visitations of Mother Mary to small clusters of openhearted devotees (as narrated through *their* devoted memoirs) allow her to bestow limitless compassion to the multitudes.

In the *Bhagavad-Gita,* Sri Krishna plays both the strict teacher and the loving, compassionate friend. The story vacillates between the harshness of fighting a righteous war and the peace of recognizing the Divine in all. It is up to the reader to choose to fight or nestle into the compassion Lord Krishna has for all his devotees.

Many examples from the Holy Scriptures tantalize us with the kind of power that comes from exerting our might and overcoming fear. Less often we are reminded that abounding in love and compassion we are led to revere, not fear, the Divine.

Mahatma Gandhi employed the principles of *Ahimsa,* which he so dearly cherished, in dealing with the foreign intruders ruling India. He inspired all the citizens of India to love their enemy. The foreign empire, confused by the unforeseen attitude, was brought to its knees. The British retreated in peace, holding Mahatma Gandhi in the highest esteem. By encasing the principles of

Ahimsa in his heart, he dearly respected even those who caused him harm. Gandhi remains a great inspiration, exemplifying compassion in the face of adversity.

"Service is not possible unless it is rooted in love and compassion. The best way to find yourself is to lose yourself in the service of others."

—*Mahatma Gandhi*

Embracing reverence and love for all (Ahimsa), *we experience oneness.*

Most often this exalted virtue of *Ahimsa* is translated simply as "nonharming" or even "nonviolence." Again we visit the idea of placing a "non" in front of a negative trait telling us what *not to do* instead of how to espouse our true nature. It implies that we are "inherently" violent and that mischief may be lurking somewhere in the background of our minds. (Often, *Yama* is translated as "restraints.") You may even be insulted by the accusation, protesting, "I do not *harm* anyone, I am not *violent*. This sutra is not meant for me!" Neither "violence" nor "harming" was implied in the Golden Age *(Sat Yuga)*, only reverence and compassion. This is where we discover the vast cavern between *not killing* or *doing harm* and embracing reverence and love. *Ahimsa* in the latter implies that our nature is to be compassionate, and when we practice *Ahimsa* fully, all living things that come into our presence experience it.

"My religion is kindness," humbly says His Holiness the Dalai Lama, a distinguished living example of *Ahimsa*.

Embracing the great virtue of *Ahimsa* brings the knowledge that each of us feels pain, joy, disappointment, love—the full spectrum of emotions. We develop an empathy with others and our individual experience becomes the experience of all.

As we open our hearts, *Ahimsa* elegantly beams reverence and love to the many facets of our life. We accept the importance of respecting all, even those who threaten or harm us physically or emotionally. Yet, the part that many of us forget is *to treat ourselves with that same reverence and love.*

The Bible compassionately tells us to "Love thy neighbor as thy self." The difficult lesson for many of us is to learn to love and serve yourself first.

Embracing reverence and love for all (Ahimsa), *we experience oneness.*

When we refuse to take the time to treat our bodies, emotions, and minds with reverence and love, they will often remind us—not so kindly—by failing to respond when we need them. Our ability to think clearly recedes. We may experience sadness or depression. After a time our lack of ease may allow disease to creep into our life. Then we are obliged to take time for ourselves. It is much more pleasant and fun to do it willingly, before any dis-ease invites itself to your life. Love for oneself is love for all.

Listen to the wisdom of your own physical heart. A mighty pump, it selflessly distributes blood throughout the body during your entire life. The heart itself first consumes the fresh oxygenated blood coming from the lungs. The heart is intuitive enough to know that it must take care of itself so it then has the fortitude to pump the blood out to oxygenate the rest of the body. It doesn't say, "Oh, the stomach seems to need the blood because it is digesting right now. I'll send it there first."

Remembering this simple illustration from the heart, we learn that in order to better serve others, we must provide for ourselves first. It is only then that we are inspired to live for the good of all.

For most of us the practice of *Ahimsa* is shown in thousands of small actions and words throughout the day. In other countries, it inspires me to observe flower garlands adorning trucks, cars, and tractors while prized cows, goats, bulls, and camels are honored with gaily colored decorations. In this way everything is beautiful and respected. We often forget that consciousness resides in every molecule, that what we put forth reflects back to us.

Embracing reverence and love for all (Ahimsa), *we experience oneness.*

EVEN A CAR HAS CONSCIOUSNESS

One time when I was traveling with Sri Swami Satchidanandaji, we were late for a *satsang* (spiritual gathering). After hastily opening the car door for him, Susan noisily slammed the door shut. Immediately, Sri Swamiji turned around and, with a look of alarm, asked her to apologize to the car. Feeling ridiculous and hoping that he was joking, she continued to walk. Sri Swamiji said, "Don't you realize what service this car has done for us? Without its assistance we would not be able to come this distance. It has brought us here safely and in comfort. For that service you, thoughtlessly, have slammed its door and caused the whole car to vibrate and be hurt." After that heartfelt explanation, Susan walked back to the car and with a gentle caress, explained how sorry she was to have slammed the door. The cars I drive, even today, still benefit from this great lesson of long ago.

Even if you inadvertently harm yourself or others, generously bathe the injury in love and compassion. *Ahimsa* is a permanent reminder for those of us determined to live each moment with the knowledge that we are all Divine.

"If you truly loved yourself, you could never hurt another."
—*Lord Buddha*

Embracing reverence and love for all (Ahimsa), *we experience oneness.*

EXPERIENCING THE JOY OF LIVING WITH REVERENCE FOR ALL *(AHIMSA)*

Ahimsa *is a vast and continuous practice. Rather than waking up tomorrow morning and vowing to have reverence for everyone and everything all the time, it is better to choose something specific and obvious. Giving yourself the opportunity to succeed is in itself* Ahimsa.

Is there a person or a situation that could assist you in your practice? Is there someone whom you have treated unkindly or who has treated you unkindly? Perhaps it was someone at the office who could be soothed by an offering of flowers or a healthy treat. Healing the hurt that already exists is a great beginning to the practice of Ahimsa.

EXPERIENCING HAVING REVERENCE FOR THE SMALL AND SIMPLE ASPECTS OF LIFE

For continuous remembrance of Ahimsa, *try embracing the simple.*

Each time you close a drawer or a door, do so with gentleness and reverence, affirming that it, too, has consciousness. Each day we close scores of drawers and doors, helping to bring Ahimsa *into the moment.*

Begin to observe the way you walk. Is your step light or heavy? Do you clunk around the house or office? Sometimes the smallest and lightest people make the loudest noises. It is not physical size; it is mental consciousness. Are you considerate of others on floors below you? Are your shoes leaving scuff marks on the floor?

When you walk outside on the grass, are you aware of all the little creatures that live in that same earth? Awareness blesses them as your foot steps softly.

Add other practices as your consciousness flourishes. Always keep Ahimsa *at the center of your thoughts, words, and actions.*

ii.36 *Dedicated to truth and integrity* (Satya), *our thoughts, words, and actions gain the power to manifest.*

Satya is a profound virtue espoused by most major traditions as a dedication to the unspoken truth that nestles in our hearts. Through *Satya* we embrace the depth of truth that words can only hope to convey.

There are many ways to access the truth. The depth of our heart's chasm measures the integrity necessary to approach real truth. The power *(shakti)* of truth is created through the alchemy of personal integrity, knowledge, and humility.

Can you "feel" truth as a physical reaction to the energy that is present, long before the mind has captured the words? Tears may fall spontaneously as your heart unfolds, ready to receive. With energy and words that dim truth, do you experience a tightening in the body that releases a wash of fear and anxiety? The heart rests when it is in *Satya*.

"Is it true? Is it kind? Is it necessary?"

—*Sufi saying*

Our words are so very powerful that we often do not realize the benefits or consequences they bestow on others or ourselves. Although our actions may appear to be benevolent, our words or thoughts may betray us with their expressions. Sometimes we misunderstand the true purpose of *Satya*.

TRUTH OR OPINION?

Walking down the street in Manhattan, I overheard a conversation: "It's too bad if she is angry with me," a woman said with indignation. "You were very harsh with her," added her kind companion. "I was just telling her *the truth!* She can't blame her hurt feelings on me!"

"Maybe what you expressed was not the truth, but *your interpretation* of the truth," her friend softly offered.

A conversation similar to this one takes place countless times a day. Often we mistake our truth for the prejudices that are formed through the colored lenses of our minds. Our words are then formed based on this formula. When our minds and hearts remain expanded, truth shines through.

As we learn to live in *Satya*, we become familiar with where integrity and truth lie. As we step into that stream, all our experiences are invited to flow along in the same direction. The more we live not just *our* version of the truth, but the truth for itself, the more the other aspects in our life neatly join the order.

Dedicated to truth and integrity (Satya), *our thoughts, words, and actions gain the power to manifest.*

"A word is a bird and the teeth are the cage; if we let the bird fly, we can never get it back."

—*Sri Swami Sivananadaji*

Getting ready to go out, your friend comes out of the bathroom and asks, "How do you like my new dress?" Withholding an audible gasp, you take a second to pause. What was she thinking to buy a dress like that? Both the color and the style are awful. She will be stared at and laughed at if she goes to the party like that. What to do?

If you tell her that you dislike the dress, you will ruin her evening. If you don't tell her how you feel, you are not living in integrity with your heart. Not a simple choice.

Take a moment to breathe deeply. As you do, remember that there were many people who thought this dress was beautiful. There was the one who designed it, the one who sewed it, the buyer at the store, and, lastly, your dear friend. Maybe, just maybe, it is your *opinion* of the dress, not the absolute truth.

"*You* look beautiful tonight, radiant as always." The decision to tell her *your* truth tomorrow saved a great deal of hurt feelings tonight.

> "Most people will not remember what you said or what you did.
> But they will remember how you made them feel."
>
> —*Maya Angelou*

Can you remember a time when you attempted to cover up a falsehood? Did it seem as though the whole world was there to expose you? At other times, when in alignment with your integrity, the potency of the truth could be felt everywhere you went.

GOSSIPING DEFUSES OUR NERVOUS SYSTEMS

The so-called "fight or flight" syndrome is considered a normal male response to a sympathetic nervous system reaction. The response is different when the same feelings are elicited in a woman's nervous system. As women, we process our stress differently from men. If there is great danger, a man's natural instinct is either to fight or to flee.

Being maternal by nature, women are engineered to protect. When danger approaches, we become quiet and still and ask our children to respond the same way. What then happens when the danger passes? We must somehow allow that internalized fear to dissipate. Men can release stress by working it out in the gym. While women receive *some* benefit from a physical release, we often find more comfort in sharing and expressing feelings with others. If this is not done, our feelings burrow deep within; sadly, this normal instinct to freeze and withdraw often leads us to depression. A woman's more verbal response to emotionally charged events has been misunderstood and criticized for ages.

The now derogatory term "gossip" originally meant "to see God" or "God-parent." Gossiping actually started as an alarm system. Women hanging clothes to dry would pass on news of the town, warnings, or any unpleasant experiences, especially with abusive men. They would whisper these messages hoping to avail others of this peril. When the men found out that their names were being dragged through the mud (or in this case the clean sheets), they decreed a severe punishment for any gossiping.

"We must not be afraid to follow the truth no matter where it may lead."
—*Thomas Jefferson*

"If in doubt whether to observe *Ahimsa* or *Satya,* always go with *Ahimsa.*"
—*Swami Vivekananda*

Dedicated to truth and integrity (Satya), *our thoughts, words, and actions gain the power to manifest.*

EXPERIENCING TRUTH AND INTEGRITY (SATYA)

Can you "feel" truth? How does it affect you when you read or hear something that you know to be true? Untrue?

Observe where on your body you feel truth and untruth.

To further enhance this practice of observation, choose an idea or a concept that you "feel" is untrue. Where is that conviction coming from? Did you ever believe it to be true?

Choose a concept that you feel is true. Where is that conviction coming from? Did you ever have any doubt?

Can you feel both truth and untruth reverberate in your body, thoughts, and feelings?

How do they then manifest in your speech and action?

How do they manifest in your life?

Do you find your integrity compromised or enhanced?

Gradually begin to trust and accept your inner knowing.

There is much in this world that will support you when you have a deep inner conviction.

11.37 *Abiding in generosity and honesty* (Astheya), *material and spiritual prosperity is bestowed.*

Our world encourages us to achieve more, amass more, and yet most of us feel we are lacking in many aspects of our life. *Astheya* has the power to initiate us into material and spiritual prosperity beyond our greatest expectations.

On a philosophical level we understand that we came into this world free of material possessions and when we leave, we leave with nothing. Even our bodies that were provided for us must stay, affirming that what we use on this earth belongs to the earth. Casually we speak about owning land or a house, yet can we move that acre of land from Montana to Florida in the winter months for warmth? It seems more like the earth is housing *us*, owning *us*.

Knowing all this, we still think of things as "mine." We attach strong possessive pronouns before objects, as if that protects us from them ever leaving us: *my* house, *her* car, *his* pen. We then become offended if someone takes something that is *mine*. We legislate to protect us from thieves, but the laws are not able to protect us from the *fear* of loss. When we don the attitude of caretakers instead of owners, we enjoy things when they come and let them go with ease. It is nature's rhythm: all things come *and* all things go.

GIVING PERMISSION TO GIVE

One of my sister monks was enjoying the water cascading down her back when she realized she forgot to bring her shampoo into the shower. Not wanting to stop, dry off, or drip water onto the floor, she pondered using *my* shampoo, which was sitting on the shelf. After silently asking my permission, she proceeded to lather up. At the same moment the image of her using my shampoo came to me. Immediately, permission was joyfully granted.

"You are always welcome to use my shampoo," I greeted her as she walked from the shower room wrapped in a towel. "How did you know?" she asked. I answered, "I felt your 'call for permission' and it was instantly given."

> "If someone asks for your shirt, give them your coat also."
> —*New Testament*

Abiding in generosity and honesty (Astheya), *material and spiritual prosperity is bestowed.*

GIVING GENEROUSLY OF ONESELF

Astheya encompasses not only generosity of money and giving of things, but also generosity of time and giving from our hearts. When you set a time for an appointment, make it a priority to be there *on time*. Otherwise you are taking energy from the person you are scheduled to meet. Your intentions may be honorable as you set your departure time, but there are always one or two quick things you could do before leaving. Oh, well, I might be *slightly* late, but that's okay, you think to yourself. That kind of thinking leads us away from an openhearted exchange. When we do meet, the beginning of the interaction is likely to be very uncomfortable. You will feel the need to apologize or explain. She will have arranged her schedule to fit this allotted time, perhaps, making sacrifices so she could be on time. When she waits for you, you become a thief, stealing her time. If this becomes a frequent occurrence, even longtime friendships can be strained. Much of the spiritual energy that you are accruing will dissipate.

Ever have the experience of reading an interesting e-mail on the computer when you are interrupted by a phone call from a distressed friend? Are you able to draw your mind from the e-mail and generously give her your full heart and mind? Or do you let her talk as you continue to be involved with the text message? Generosity gives great gifts in many small ways.

In the face of great tragedy, people are known to open their hearts to those considered strangers just minutes before. Others needing an outlet for their pain and frustration may intentionally snatch any remnants of calm they feel from others.

After the catastrophic events of September 11, 2001, the devastation continued as many sought to blame and punish the perpetrators of this heinous crime. In lieu of a healthy outlet, their frustrations continued to be fueled by the inability to locate the agitators. Feelings of helplessness stoked the rage as it burst out, scorching an innocent population. The wave of hatred overtook and stole what little safety was left in many ethnic communities guilty of nothing more than having the same religious background or national origin as the terrorists.

For most parents the original disaster was difficult enough to explain to their children. They were now grasping for whatever goodness they could gather to protect the innocence of their children and to calm the colossal fear. Humbly they sought the sage advice of one of the icons of kindheartedness in the world of children. Mr. Rogers, a longtime TV host and minister, encouraged and empowered countless children to live with kindness and love. His advice whispers the secret of generosity from time immemorial: "Tell the children to watch the helpers. Their generosity of heart and time is an inspiration to us all. It can help soothe our pain as it encourages our hearts to open."

Abiding in generosity and honesty (Astheya), *material and spiritual prosperity is bestowed.*

The vibration of *Astheya* magnifies our experience of prosperity, smoothing the way for us to give generously to others. At times when our hearts are open, generosity cascades unencumbered. At other times, we must recall when we were bathed in our own generosity or that of another, and how blessed we felt.

In our lives we have many occasions to give. In the simplest way, *Astheya* tells us not to steal. As it expands your heart, it says, *give*. For maximum benefit, do not even wait for someone to ask, be alert, and never miss an opportunity to give, give, give. Sri Swami Sivanandaji's students who hoped to emulate his most generous nature gave him the nickname of Swami Give-*ananda* (the bliss of giving).

> "To believe in something, and not to live it, is dishonest."
> —*Mahatma Gandhi*

Abiding in generosity and honesty (Astheya), *material and spiritual prosperity is bestowed.*

EXPERIENCING THE GRACE OF GENEROSITY AND HONESTY (*ASTHEYA*)

Observe your life, and with a generous heart envision the great and small ways you experience wealth and prosperity. Make a list. The list may include the bounty of food you have access to whenever you feel hunger, or your closet filled with clothes for all types of weather and conditions and events.

Notice if your comfort expands to giving generously to others. Or do you still feel you need more before you can do that?

From the material, move toward generosity of time. Are you always ready to greet others and be helpful? Do you keep others waiting? Can you stop what you are doing to respect the other person's schedule?

Observe the way your heart can be generous in giving service to others.

In what ways are you generous with yourself? Do you take the time to nurture yourself on all levels?

In what small ways can you expand your generosity on a daily basis? As your generosity expands, your heart's capacity to give will increase incrementally.

II.38 *Devoted to living a balanced and moderate life* (Brahmacharya), *the scope of one's life force becomes boundless.*

Our journey through the *Yamas* is reminding us to blend our human and Divine nature by reflecting reverence for all *(Ahimsa)* and living in truth *(Satya)* and generosity *(Astheya)*. We are now introduced to the concept of moderation and balance, *Brahmacharya*. Through this practice we are able to orchestrate the glorious dance between our Divine nature and human nature. Each is fueled by the vital energy that is generated as we emulate, rather than resist, nature's beautiful patterns.

DON'T UPSET MOTHER NATURE!

When nature's balance is upset and large amounts of energy are deployed at one time, the repercussions can be devastating. A raging forest fire, a hurricane, a blizzard, a volcanic eruption, an earthquake:

all are dynamic yet destructive releases of nature's power. Fortunately, these flare-ups are infrequent, and most of the time we enjoy nature's changes with metronome regularity, such as night and day, summer and winter, sun and rain.

Our bodies, minds, and emotions also respond positively to regular cycles and schedules. If we are fortunate, balance and moderation frame our lives, and very little of our vital energy is spent making adjustments or restoring equilibrium.

Brahmacharya, the art of living a moderate life, is a challenging practice in our modern society. When times were simpler, we were more aware and respectful of our bodies, minds, and emotions. The need to adjust our energy was heeded before our energy was depleted ("before" is key). A farmer, knowingly or unknowingly, designs her or his lifestyle according to the fluctuations of nature's cycles. During the planting and harvest time, s/he understands that a large outpouring of energy is necessary. The respite needed to replenish the weary body will come naturally with the shorter days and longer nights of winter. The rhythm of the seasons *naturally* restores balance.

In these modern times, because of great technological advances, our activities no longer depend on times of day or the seasons. We have the ability to control heat and cold, light and darkness. Manipulating nature in this way seems to encourage everything *but* moderation. The concept of moderation is usurped by the "do more and then do much more" attitude. If our tendency is toward over-activity, society waves our speeding train onward. The ability to earn an income while living a life of balance seems more difficult in these contemporary times.

RESPECTING OUR VITAL ENERGY

Relating to vital energy is similar to the way we relate to our monetary energy. If I have $100 in my bank account, then that is the most I should spend. If I spent the entire $100, then I would technically not have any more money to spend. However, if I decide to spend $100 and borrow another $50, I would not just be depleted; I would now be in debt. If this continues, I might borrow more to pay off the loan and go deeper into debt. With this large depletion, how is it possible to generate *more* to pay back what I owe?

Translating this way of thinking back to our own personal energy, if we live in moderation, we have plenty of energy to spend. We can spend it in many ways. Some can go into service, some for fun and pleasure, and there will still be plenty available for our spiritual practices. If we overspend our portion of energy and go into debt, the vitality and vigor needed for spiritual practice will be unavailable.

We all know the feeling after eating a big holiday dinner. Our belly is so stuffed full of food we are only able to lie on the couch, groaning. Even for the next few days, we will feel exhausted and lethargic, having overdrawn our energy account trying to digest and assimilate the enormous quantity of food. Experiencing this discomfort, we then tend to swing to the other extreme and eat too little. This depletes the vitality and strength needed to nourish the mind, emotions, and body. Only when the physical realm is in a state of balance is there ample energy to drive us to the more subtle spiritual vistas.

Overeating is only *one* of the ways we expend this energy. All of our senses can be enablers. Too much TV, computer work, even reading will draw on and deplete our vital force. Extreme physical exercise may leave us feeling exhausted. Too frequent sexual activity without emotional content causes depletion. Listening to very loud music or talking too much all create an energetic liability. For our life force to remain strong and available, *all* aspects of our lives need to be balanced.

"Yoga is not for one who eats too much, or for one who fasts too much, nor sleeps too much or sleeps too little, but instead lives in a harmonious flow along the middle path."

—*Bhagavad-Gita*

Devoted to living a balanced and moderate life (Brahmacharya), *the scope of one's life force becomes boundless.*

THE POWER OF SEXUAL ENERGY

If *Brahmacharya* is meant to convey a sense of balance and moderation in our life, why is it usually translated as celibacy or continence?

About the time the sutras and other holy books of India were being translated into English, much of Western Europe was enmeshed in a puritanical mind-set. This influenced their interpretation of the Bible, which then manipulated their outlook on life.

This mind-set brought with it explicit doctrine prohibiting any sexual expression in thought, word, or action. (It was allowed only for procreation, and no one had better enjoy it!) Repressing sexual expression caused monumental adverse effects both on physical health and on emotional stability. The women became the evil courtesans enticing innocent men to act against God. Remember, this was the time when women were persecuted for being women! Even with all the guilt and apprehension, the human species continued to reproduce, unconcerned about fundamentalist doctrine.

The Western religious fundamentalists living in India felt it their hallowed duty to impose the same puritanical values on their hosts' way of life. The restrictions were reflected both in the secular and religious realms.

WOMAN AS TEMPTRESS

Of course the *women* of India were targeted, and a decree to alter their way of dressing was issued. For thousands of years, the traditional dress was a sari. Many yards of unsewn fabric were wound around the waist, covering the lower part of the body, and the last two yards were draped over one shoulder. This afforded them enough modesty and was very practical for breastfeeding. But the idea that a woman's breast would be so readily available was a disgraceful thought to the foreigners. Women were taught how to sew (a nonexistent art in India before this time) in order that blouses could be made to cover and hide their breasts. If you venture into the remote villages even today, you will see women who escaped this edict.

> "India lives in her villages."
>
> —*Indira Gandhi*

We often are very unsophisticated in thinking that what is acceptable behavior in one country or district is acceptable throughout the world. This is especially apparent in what we consider moral and appropriate sexual behavior. If it is not your belief, it may be difficult to reconcile yourself with the fact that—in some parts of the world—it is permissible to take on many husbands or wives. In some places you can take on one or more of each!

In the opening scene of John Patrick and Vern Sneider's *Tea House of the August Moon,* a very distinguished Japanese gentleman appears alone on stage. He bows and begins to address the audience of Americans. "In *our* country taking bath with strange naked lady *is* socially acceptable. Hanging picture of strange naked lady on living room wall is *not* socially acceptable. In *your* country taking bath with strange naked lady *is not* acceptable. Hanging picture of strange naked lady on living room wall *is* acceptable. Therefore, my friends, you see, *pornography is simply a matter of geography!"*

Devoted to living a balanced and moderate life (Brahmacharya), **the scope of one's life force becomes boundless.**

For millennia, yogis who knew the importance of balance, moderation, and redirecting sexual energy developed specific practices for this purpose. They understood that we, like all of nature, ebb and flow through cycles, sometimes needing to use our sexual energy and other times to preserve it. With the surge of puritanical Western thinking, the dignity of moderation and balance became distorted. This repression caused a rise in celibacy, driving many of the sacred teachings underground. The path of celibacy was then elevated as the zenith of spirituality and the quickest way to reach the Divine.

One of the most detrimental consequences of this misinterpretation was the separation of spirit from nature. Women (representing nature) were rejected from spiritual communion. Up to this time, the woman was seen as the *shakti* (manifesting energy) without whom the man could not function!

EXPLORING THE FOUR *ASHRAMAS,* OR STAGES, OF LIFE

According to the ancient ways, there were four stages of life that one passed through, learning a variety of lessons and experiences in each. They offered an expanding way of service to one's self, one's family, the spiritual community (*satsang*), and the entire world.

Living in balance, each individual had a life span of one hundred years or more. It was considered to be the effect of using the life force wisely. Divided into four, each stage affords us the attributes and temperament befitting our development. While the exact span of years in each of the stages may vary, notice how they portray the yearning to change focus as we progress through life. Even practicing them inwardly propels us toward spiritual freedom.

Brahmacharya A time celebrated for creativity, play, and study. This all-important time is spent gaining knowledge about your relationship to your self, the world, and the Divine. It is a time to explore and set patterns as to where and how you want to direct your energy. Because it is not yet the time for intimate relationships, as sexual energy begins to mature, the vital energy is available for study and learning and introspection.

Ghrihasta The time has come to explore the world and all her abundant gifts. Settling on a profession or trade, you now embrace a long-term loving relationship. The refined vital sexual energy that has been cherished is available in its wholesome form to lovingly pleasure another, and to create and nurture children.

Vanaprasta Less time is spent on your profession; the children are grown and have children of their own. You and your partner still enjoy physical intimacy and find the earlier intensity has evolved into deep tenderness and devotion. As more leisure time is available, you long to spend it in spiritual practice and study.

Sannyasa Letting go of worldly duties and desires, you are drawn more toward the spiritual than the physical world. Drawing inward, most of your treasured time is dedicated to service, study, and devotion of the Divine.

As we can see, the four *Ashramas* of life seemed to follow a very natural and productive pattern. Each person transitioned through the various stages in the order presented. Spirituality was never intended to be a separate addition to life; it *was* life. As one reached the *Sannyasa* phase of withdrawing from the world, it was as natural as a snake shedding its skin. Occasionally, a few men (and only men at the time) were called to renounce personal life at an earlier age. They would then choose to remain unmarried, thus allowing them to be free to serve all without prejudice or favor.

For centuries the origin of women's power has been a mystery to men, and they have done much to try to capture it though repression, possession, and various tedious sexual practices. As we respect and esteem the vital energy, we are humbled to realize it holds the power to create another human being.

If abstinence were the sure way to the Divine, many people throughout the world would be realized beings. Like so many practices, it is more in the essence than in the act. Engage in the pleasures of making love as *Karma Yoga*. Your only desire is to pleasure the other person, and their only desire is to pleasure you. Each is fulfilled and satisfied, and when we are satisfied, we are moderate and balanced.

Devoted to living a balanced and moderate life (Brahmacharya), *the scope of one's life force becomes boundless.*

EXPERIENCING MODERATION (*BRAHMACHARYA*) IN YOUR LIFE

Are there certain areas in your life where you could be more moderate? It could be food, work, TV, and so on. Choose one at a time and begin to moderate its use. For this example we will use food.

If you are accustomed to eating three large meals a day and many snacks, begin to eat less at meal times and half as much when you snack. Instead of two handfuls of nuts, take one.

The tendency would be to eat only one meal and eliminate all snacks. That would swing the pendulum from one extreme to the other. Remember, the idea is to practice moderation. We already know how to be excessive!

Notice how much energy you feel after a few days.

Then you can progress to moderating TV watching or working too long.

Slowly begin to move though all the areas in your life until moderation is the norm.

II.39 *Acknowledging abundance* (Aparigraha), *we recognize the blessings in everything and gain insights into the purpose for our worldly existence.*

Aparigraha gives us the secret to earthly life. Take a moment to feel gratitude for the great blessings that surround you: the home you live in, the service you do in the world, the availability and quantity of food you have to eat. The riches also include your friends, your health, and the opportunity to dedicate time to know your own heart. Even when you acknowledge the bounty, is there still a lingering apprehension that part or all of it may be taken away? That the well might run dry? Just thinking that a resource is limited initiates fear, thereby lessening the joy in the present moment.

As a society, we enjoy luxuries that were not even awarded to the royalty of the past. They were not blessed with the simple comforts we now consider everyday requirements. Central heat and air-conditioning, indoor plumbing, or simply a knob to turn in order to cook our meals are often taken for granted. The next time you are called to nature in the middle of the night, be thankful it is as near as the next heated room.

As a nation, our facade of abundance is possible because of what we imaginatively call credit, which in reality is debt. Debt is what we *really* accumulate when we amass all the so-called necessities we could not possibly live without. This masquerade is facilitated by our engorged belief in propriety and greed. Creating a complex misunderstanding of the flow of abundance, we tend to overlook the premise that when money is owed, obligation is accrued. Most importantly, we have distracted ourselves from the true happiness within by impeding the access into the spiritual vistas with material wants and needs. If we are able to live within the material energy allotted us and generously use the word "Enough," abundance cascades in our direction. We become free.

LET GO AND BE FREE

We all know and recite the phrase "Money cannot buy happiness," yet we often trade our peace and health for the material security necessary to sustain our escalating lifestyle. Spiritual wealth is the only wealth that sustains us and when we venture deep within, we are all millionaires!

Life's ebb and flow brings things into our life and then out again. Even the slightest hesitation of holding impedes the flow. Our belief system has the ability to hinder or expand this flow of abundance. If you believe that material and spiritual blessings are infinite, a cornucopia awaits you. If, instead, you accept the bounty as limited, your hopes and dreams will shrink to those proportions.

Our habit of waste runs contradictory to *Aparigraha*. If we really believed that this was our *last* meal, would we not savor the food we have on our plate? In our fear of not getting enough, we often take too much on our plates only to throw away the leftovers. As a nation, we are great consumers, and also great wasters. We may buy a dress for one occasion and never wear it again, but keep it *just in case.* Or every few years we might buy a new car that is bigger than the last, with an engine that consumes greater quantities of fossil fuels. How much does this affect us?

> "If we shut our ears to the cry of the poor, we may also cry out
> and not be answered."
>
> —*Proverb*

Some allow material possessions to easily come and go; it is their thoughts and ideas that are etched in stone. When you form an opinion of someone or something, how effortlessly can you allow that opinion to change? One of the most difficult things is for us to change our thoughts and ways. Even more difficult is for us to accept the change in others.

> "What is it that you lost that you are grieving for? What is it that you
> brought into this world that you have lost? Whatever you gained, you
> gained from this world. Whatever you lost, you lost to this world. What
> belongs to you today, belonged to someone else yesterday and will
> belong to someone else tomorrow."
>
> —*Bhagavad-Gita*

Acknowledging abundance (Aparigraha), *we recognize the blessings in everything and gain insights into the purpose for our worldly existence.*

EXPERIENCING ABUNDANCE (*APARIGRAHA*) BY LETTING THINGS GO

Clean out a drawer or a closet and give the contents to a worthy person or charity. An empty place allows for new things to abundantly fill your life.

Move this same idea to your date book. Leave some time each week for the unexpected to happen. Invite surprise blessings to visit you.

EXPERIENCING GRATITUDE FOR YOUR ABUNDANCE (*APARIGRAHA*)

Plan some time, perhaps at the holidays, to feed the homeless or to read to the sick or the elderly.

Notice and record any mental or emotional resistance.

Review the way you live your life and try to imagine for what purpose you are here on this earth.

Note how you feel after the experience.

Do you feel an expansiveness and an experience of gratitude that accompanies it? Perhaps so much so, that you may want to make this kind of Seva (Selfless Service) a regular event in your life.

NIYAMA:
Evolution Toward Harmony

FIVE INNER FACETS of *Asthaanga Yoga* are presented here as *Niyama,* allowing us to continue our journey inward toward wholeness and discovering our divinity.

Through simplicity and continual refinement (Saucha),
the body, thoughts, and emotions become clear reflections
of the Self within.

Saucha reveals our joyful nature, and the yearning
for knowing the Self blossoms.

When at peace and content with oneself and others
(Santosha), supreme joy is celebrated.

Living life with zeal and sincerity, the purifying flame is
ignited (Tapas), revealing the inner light.

Sacred study of the Divine through scripture,
nature, and introspection (Swadhaya) guides us
to the Supreme Self.

Through wholehearted dedication (Iswara Pranidhana),
we become intoxicated with the Divine.

11.40 *Through simplicity and continual refinement* (Saucha), *the body, thoughts, and emotions become clear reflections of the Self within.*

11.41 Saucha *reveals our joyful nature, and the yearning for knowing the Self blossoms.*

Through the practice of *Saucha* our flawless essence becomes the basis for the choices and directions we invite into our life.

Pure silver is a lucid and shiny metal. Unrefined, it appears ordinary, its luminescence hidden. The process requires the silversmith to boil the unrefined silver over the hottest flame. It is essential for her to fully attend to the molten silver during this tedious process. If the silver remains in the fire for a moment longer than necessary, it could be destroyed. The correct amount of time yields awesome beauty. How does the silversmith know when the silver is fully refined? When she can clearly see her image in it.

Saucha recalls the simple and pure energy of youth that fostered healthy development on all levels of our being. The same longing for simplicity, though sometimes hindered, continues throughout our lifetime.

PURIFICATION BY NATURE

Many cultures have ritualistic bathing practices to encourage the continuation of this lifelong refinement. Early-morning immersions in a holy river, often performed while repeating prayers, purify not only the body but the mind and emotions as well, so the light in the heart can be experienced. Baptism purifies the body so the blessed spirit within can shine. On a less esoteric level, the enrichment gained by soaking in a natural hot spring, sauna, or steam bath continues to delight many throughout the ages.

Women's bodies naturally cycle through their own unique phases—ovulation, menstruation, conception, pregnancy, childbirth, menopause. These dramatic sequences symbolize the highly sophisticated ways our bodies stay vital and healthy. Unable to understand the purpose for these cleansing cycles, male authority figures distorted them, marking women unclean and tainted during "certain times of the month." Firm rules were established to keep us from "contaminating" men or sacred objects. Rituals were devised to purify and sanitize us before we could be accepted into the larger society again.

Yet was that not the job our bodies had just completed? The act of menstruating itself is purification! Driven by natural forces, we are *different* from men, not tarnished or unclean. All this ostracism could have been avoided with the alluring knowledge that the only true purity is *in each heart*. We were framed by a misconception so great that even today, women are thought to be unclean during those "special" times!

> "Respect woman as my equal in creation as bearing the image of God."
> —*The Bible*

Through simplicity and continual refinement (Saucha), *the body, thoughts, and emotions become clear reflections of the Self within.*

Saucha *reveals our joyful nature, and the yearning for knowing the Self blossoms.*

EVERYTHING IS HOLY TO THOSE WITH AN OPEN HEART

Nurses are the angels of mercy in the medical profession. They serve with compassion, and take their rewards from knowing they bring comfort and healing to us. Often they have the unpleasant duty of cleaning up bodily discharges. It is their purity of heart that allows them to serve us at our greatest and most humbling time of need without judgment or aversion.

The illustrious Florence Nightingale formalized the nursing profession. Abandoning her privilege and status, she chose to dedicate her life to the sick and infirm. The essence of compassion, "the lady with the lamp" selflessly spent long hours bringing comfort to many. She revolutionized hospital care with simple yet essential improvements. Basic procedures we now take for granted, such as keeping the body washed and dressings clean and placing a bell at the bedside, allotted patients dignity in the face of distress.

Mother Teresa of Calcutta many years later exemplified Florence Nightingale's basic principles. Encountering the destitute and the sick lying on the streets, she cradled them in her arms, impervious to the unsanitary conditions of their bodies, offering them "a moment of love and dignity before they died."

When difficulties would arise during our Healing Retreats for those with cancer, Mother Teresa's words returned to inspire me: "The miracle is not that we do this work. The miracle is that we *love* to do this work."

NOT-SO-OBVIOUS SIMPLICITY

Cultivating simplicity of mind and emotions can be a refreshing change from the complicated world we live in.

When American scientists were making plans to send the first human into weightless space, they encountered many challenges that gravity-bound Earth did not have. Something as routine as keeping a log facilitated the invention of a special writing instrument. In normal usage, ink flows downward from the pen to the paper. This is all done with the persistent force of gravity. Without this force, the ink floats any which way, making writing impossible. Finally, millions of dollars in research and development yielded a pen that could do the job of writing in zero gravity. The ship's logs could now be filled in. The Russians, however, took the simpler route and saved an enormous amount of money. They used a pencil!

It is truly a "gift to be simple." The blessings come when we can embrace simplicity, making our lives easier and more joyous. *Saucha* is the purity deep within our own heart that resonates as our guide to knowing.

> "Blessed are the pure in Heart for they shall know God."
>
> —*New Testament Bible*

Another aspect of *Saucha* is the ability to be emotionally light. We tend to take situations and ourselves much too seriously. Observing the humor in life promotes emotional purity.

> "The Divine is the only Comedian, playing to an audience
> who has forgotten how to laugh."
>
> —*Voltaire*

Through simplicity and continual refinement (Saucha), *the body, thoughts, and emotions become clear reflections of the Self within.*

Saucha *reveals our joyful nature, and the yearning for knowing the Self blossoms.*

EXPERIENCING THE POWER OF PURITY AND SIMPLICITY (*SAUCHA*)

Observe how your body changes with the different foods you eat. If the weather is hot and you eat spicy or warming foods, notice if your body perspires more than it does when you consume cool foods or drinks.

When watching a scary movie or reading a disturbing book, notice how your thoughts and emotions mimic that mood. It could be an immediate response, or it could be a delayed one in a totally different situation.

Are there certain clothes or surroundings that allow you to feel a sense of refinement in your being?

When you walk on a pristine beach, or in a forest, does the simplicity of nature afford the mind and emotions a joyful feeling? Does it seem like all the worries you brought with you surrender to the peaceful surroundings?

Write down which foods, clothes, and places allow you to feel that sense of purity, simplicity, and refinement. How do they assist you in feeling that way? The next time you are deciding what to eat, what to wear, or where to visit, recall what feeling you want to invoke and then follow its lead in choosing.

When you are involved in a stressful situation, try to look at it from another way, finding a bit of humor that can lighten the mood. Laughter allows the heart to blossom.

II.42 *When at peace and content with oneself and others* (Santosha), *supreme joy is celebrated.*

Santosha is an agreement of faith that we make with our Divine Self. This faith fastens us to the peace that abides in our hearts, no matter what the fates bring. By this affirmation we firmly identify with our inner essence rather than with external objects. Our identification then travels with gratitude, appreciating how much we have rather than how much we want. With this attitude, all things that come and go do not have the opportunity to override our joy. Instead, they metamorphose into stillness and peace.

KEEPING YOUR HEART LIGHT AS A FEATHER

In ancient Egypt, after death, the heart was removed from the body to be measured against the weight of a feather. If the heart was found to be heavier than the feather's weight, the person was considered not ready for admission to heaven. The scale, although normally the measure of physical weight, was thought to reveal the degree of emotional heaviness held in the heart. The *lighthearted* were presumably permitted entry through a special ritual, as their physical heart was given a place of honor in the burial plot.

> "Content with an ordinary life, you can show all people
> the way back to their own true nature."
>
> —*Lao-tzu*

When at peace and content with oneself and others (**Santosha**), *supreme joy is celebrated.*

JOY IS ACCEPTING WHAT IS

Some of us open naturally to joy, while others need to cultivate it more carefully. For most of us, the subtler aspects of *Santosha* elude us from time to time. Everlasting joy cleaves to us through cultivating the understanding that we hold the power to our happiness. Even if temporarily lost, our joy will soon return, as it is the lifelong reward for attaining wisdom.

In South India there is a heartfelt way of expressing one's appreciation. Instead of saying "thank you," they say "*Santosha* [I am content]."

When at peace and content with oneself and others (Santosha), supreme joy is celebrated.

EXPERIENCING YOUR JOYFUL NATURE

Venture to a comfortable place, either physically or in your imagination, where the surroundings evoke a feeling of peace and joy.

Spend a few minutes experiencing comfort with the ambiance and notice if you spontaneously begin to smile.

Once the smile forms, let it engrave on your face, close the eyes, and journey inward.

Notice how the outer smile is greeted by the inner smile of contentment in your heart.

The smile is the outward expression of the joy.

When you leave the physical place that invoked this feeling, the outward smile remains as the constant reminder of your inner contentment. Sharing it with each person you meet is like sharing a place in your heart.

*If at any time the contentment seems to be hiding, coax it out
with a sweet upturning of your lips and cheeks and a sparkle in
your eyes.*

II.43 *Living life with zeal and sincerity, the purifying flame is ignited* (Tapas), *revealing the inner light.*

Once again we visit *Tapas, Swadhaya,* and *Iswara Pranidhana,* which
complemented each other as *Kriya Yoga,* Sutra II. 1. This time they
are woven into *Asthaanga Yoga,* as the final three *Niyamas.* Their
importance is reinforced by their repetition in the *sutras.*

TAPAS OF BODY, MIND, AND SPEECH

The *Bhagavad-Gita* speaks to us of *Tapas,* kindling the purifying
flame through refining the actions of our bodies, minds, and speech.
   Tapas of Body is defined as service, physical purity, living in
virtue, moderation, and reverence for all.
   Charging all your actions with zeal and sincerity—whether serving family, the greater community, or yourself—transforms them
into spiritual practice. This concept applies to the formal practices
as well. When practicing asana (posture), *pranayama* (guidance of
universal energy), or any of the other practices, the main benefit
comes from embracing the deep spiritual intention.
   Tapas of Mind is distinguished as tranquil, gentle, kind, quiet,
willpower, and purity of thought.
   How we think and feel is a predictor of our physical health and
vitality. Our relationships with the world around us are molded by

the way we *imagine* them to be. By keeping our mind tranquil, gentle, and pure, we create a life worthy of spiritual reflection.

Tapas of Speech is experienced as truthful, pleasant, serene, beneficial, prayer, and *japa* (repetition of a mantra).

Speech is a direct outward expression of the mind and emotions. If we are agitated or upset, our language mimics that point of view. Consciously choosing words that are pleasant and serene, we are able to *influence* the mind and emotions into calmness. Prayer and mantra are ways of extending the vistas of our speech to reach the place where all understanding resides.

This clear, threefold description of *Tapas* from the *Bhagavad-Gita* allows us the liberty to experience varied ways of transforming energy. When the practices are not separate from but incorporated into our lives, the unfolding of our hearts continues. The *Bhagavad-Gita* assures us that it is not necessary to engage in rigorous practices; these steady and subtle ways slowly ignite the spark of Divinity within our heart.

While there are varied forms of sacrifice one can make with zeal and sincerity, simple acts of devotion, whether private or public, have powerful and lasting effects.

Living life with zeal and sincerity, the purifying flame is ignited (Tapas), *revealing the inner light.*

AN EXQUISITE TEST OF FAITH

The brilliant poet Maya Angelou talks with passion and tenderness of one of her fiercest tests and how she ascended to a high level of understanding through sacred prayer. (This story beautifully illustrates the perfect blending of *Tapas, Swadhaya,* and *Iswara Pranidhana.*)

An alarming phone call revealed that her precious son was hospitalized and not expected to live. "Could you come quickly?" the frightened voice asked. She could hardly have arrived more quickly if she had the power to materialize at will.

The doctors were confident that her son would live only a short time longer. Hearing that proclamation, she enjoined everyone concerned to convey *only positive thoughts* when entering her son's hospital room. Summoning all her faith and strength, she began a prayer vigil that, she vowed, would continue until her son had made *a total recovery.* She would consider no other outcome. Her heart and soul entwined in chorus, "God, I am thanking you in advance for the full recovery of my son." Her prayer was clear and simple, leaving not even a hair's breadth for doubt or confusion.

Moving from the seed in her heart, the prayer flooded her mind, giving it voice. "God, I am thanking you in advance for the full recovery of my son." Over and over she prayed, in a heart-wrenching refrain that summoned compassion from all the angels, "God, I am thanking you in advance for the full recovery of my son." All through the night, aware of nothing else, her powerful voice echoed through the room and up to the heavens. Drawn by her sincerity and passion, many joined her in chorus, "God, I am thanking you in advance for the full recovery of my son." As others tired and left, she continued until she *knew* that the prayers were being heard. "God, I am thanking you in advance for the full recovery of my son." At times her voice started to waver, but never her heart.

Not until her son returned from the coma to a semiwaking state did she even begin to slow down her vigil. After the full recovery of her son, she was asked if she ever doubted that her prayers would be answered. "If doubt even started to peek its head up, I'd bellow even louder. The Good Lord might have been busy and I wanted to make sure He could hear me. And I kept the prayer going for weeks after. I was not satisfied until my son *fully recovered.*"

"I have an inward treasure born within me, which can keep me alive
if all the extraneous delights should be withheld: or offered
only at a price I cannot afford."

—*Charlotte Brontë*

Living life with zeal and sincerity, the purifying flame is ignited
(Tapas), *revealing the inner light.*

EXPERIENCING LIVING YOUR LIFE WITH ZEAL AND SINCERITY

Choose the Tapas of Speech *from the* Bhagavad-Gita *as the focus of your practice. Notice how your voice resonates and observe the choice of words you use.*

For a revealing look at this, take a small recording device and place it under a table or out of sight the next time you visit with a friend. Turn it on at the onset of your conversation. Soon you will forget it is there.

After your friend leaves, listen to your words and expressions. Was your speech tranquil and gentle? Did it bring benefit to yourself and your friend?

How was the tone of your voice? Did you feel soothed or agitated listening to yourself?

Was it enlightening to listen to yourself speaking (if perhaps a bit intimidating)?

Incorporate the positive changes you would like to introduce into your speech for a week and repeat the process.

Continue refining and, after some time, you will find the outer speech reflects not only the mind and emotions but your heart as well.

11.44 *Sacred study of the Divine through scripture, nature, and introspection* (Swadhaya) *guides us to the Supreme Self.*

Swadhaya guides us to know our selves through outward observation *and* inner reflection. Often we experience an incomprehensible phenomenon, either in nature or within our minds and hearts. If we are unable to understand it intuitively, we seek external sources. If, for example, we seek understanding of the movements of the tides or the cycles of the moon, we may consult an astronomer and conduct a thorough investigation of how gravity works.

However, if seeking a spiritual understanding, finding an outside source becomes a more delicate matter. It may take days, weeks, or longer to find a holy book or a teacher to assuage doubts or endorse experiences. Why is it we are able to learn so much from some people and have great difficulty learning from others? Is it their ability to quote great teachings or the grace they exude that transports us to the depth of understanding, or perhaps something deeper still?

One such great teacher, a revered and noble rabbi, had breathed his last breath, leaving the congregation in soulful mourning. An outsider became curious about this esteemed rabbi who drew such veneration on his death. He began interviewing a few of the close disciples who were blessed to study with the rabbi. The refrains were varied and vague. "I cannot exactly say how he inspired me; we learned the teachings through his discourses, but more was transmitted by the way he lived his life." "He was a very humble man." One disciple sitting off by himself, his eyes brimming with tears, whispered softly, "I used to love to watch the way, with great reverence, he took off his shoes."

"Study brings us wisdom, wisdom brings us life."
—Rabbi Hillel

We tend to revere book learning in these times, overstuffing our minds with all kinds of information. If you read one issue of the Sunday New York Times cover to cover, you have exposed yourself to more information than the average person one hundred years ago read during her or his entire lifetime!

FACT TODAY, FICTION TOMORROW

We often forget that observing natural occurrences has made many important discoveries. Alexander Fleming's curiosity led him to study a simple mold, offensive to most of us, making the intuitive leap that these organisms could miraculously cure infection. Commonly known as penicillin, the minute spores became the panacea that saved millions of lives.

Many theories may be correct and accurate today, but tomorrow, with new discoveries and advancements, those "truths" of yesterday may be discounted. What happens to our belief in the first theory? Is it shaken? The mind wants to switch to the new hypothesis, but how quickly are we able to change?

Several hundred years ago, a few noble scientists, including Giordano Bruno, proclaimed that the earth was not the center of the planetary system, let alone the universe! The repercussions were uproarious, and the theory was considered blasphemous. It was a well-known *fact* at that time that the sun as well as all the other planets orbited around the earth! The outraged church declared the discovery to be heresy. Bruno, a prominent astronomer, a seer, and a speaker of truth, was burned at the stake.

Later, Galileo corroborated Bruno's theory and was sentenced to house arrest for the remainder of his life. Today the knowledge that the earth revolves around the sun is a straightforward observation (we even call it the solar system), a statement of fact, but at that time the opposite was considered *truth*.

We all agree that the earth revolves around the sun; yet, we continue to use archaic language. What words do you use to describe what you observe at dawn and dusk? Do you say the sun *rises* in the morning and *sets* in the evening? Most people do. Yet, we just clearly established that the sun does not revolve around us, so how could it rise and set? Even with correct knowledge, we are slow to change our consciousness and our metaphors.

Always be willing for your concept of reality to change as your consciousness brightens.

Sacred study of the Divine through scripture, nature, and intro-spection (Swadhaya) *guides us to the Supreme Self.*

EXPERIENCING THE ROTATION OF THE EARTH AND CHANGING YOUR CONCEPT OF SUNRISE AND SUNSET

Sit or stand comfortably with a clear view of the sky at predawn or predusk.

Observe the sun and notice how your mind travels to the customary yet erroneous relationship between the sun and the earth. While your deep thoughts hold the truth, the habitual mind holds the notion that the sun rises and sets, while you, planted on the earth, remain stationary.

Become very quiet and begin to imagine that you and the earth are actually moving either toward the sun (dawn) or away from the sun (dusk). Notice how your mind will try to resist this phenomenon.

After a time, you may be able to feel the steady, slow motion. You may even get a bit dizzy.

It may take a while, but as you repeat this observation, the flow will seem more natural. Then the challenge will be to come up with other terminology for the earth's movements, letting go of the terms "sunrise" and "sunset."

Use the same principles with other concepts that you may believe to be so.

Look to a learned source for affirmation and challenge yourself to change!

II.45 *Through wholehearted dedication* (Iswara Pranidhana), *we become intoxicated with the Divine.*

For the third time in the sacred sutras, *Iswara Pranidhana* is encouraging us to live with wholehearted devotion to the Divine and Divine creation. As *Ahimsa* is the pinnacle from which all of the *Yamas* flow, *Iswara Pranidhana* is the zenith of the *Niyamas*.

Devotion is the key to unlocking our hearts. When living with an open heart, we see clearly as the pathways of our lives unfold. Faith allows us to trust in the present moment as we observe our part in the Divine plan.

Love and devotion can be expressed as a simple blessing we bestow on ourselves or others, such as saying "Bless you" when someone sneezes. Often prayers invoke a higher source for something as mundane as losing our keys: "Please, Divine Mother, help me find my keys."

MANY WAYS TO PRAY TO THE ONE

Prayers come in as many forms as there are hearts to recite them. Here are a few of the more traditional ways prayer is summoned:

Petition: appeals to the Divine to fulfill our needs or wishes (*"Divine Mother, please help me get this job."*).

Intercession: pleas made on behalf of another (*"Divine Mother, please let my daughter get into college."*).

Thanksgiving: expressions of deep gratitude (*"Thank you, Divine Mother, for allowing our home to be saved from the fire."*).

Praise: glorification of the Divine and creation (*"Blessed be You who made this beautiful day."*).

Blessings: invoking the Divine Grace to bless, protect, and guide us and others (*"Divine Mother, please bless and protect our family through this time of great trial."*).

Affirmation: heartfelt expression to the uncertainty of our faith in the Divine plan of the Universe (*"Divine Mother, I do not understand why this great sorrow is upon us; please give me the faith and strength to withstand it and keep my trust in You strong."*).

> "More things are wrought by prayer than this world dreams of."
> —*Alfred, Lord Tennyson*

Through wholehearted dedication (**Iswara Pranidhana**), *we become intoxicated with the Divine.*

Prayers can be directed to the Divine within or to an outward presence. Much of the time we go back and forth according to the moment and mood. Most of us summon the greatest power of prayer in difficult times. When all other avenues have been exhausted and the enormity of the situation becomes too great to bear alone, we then pray to someone else out there as a separate person or manifestation to help us cope. We are really just summoning all the positive energy and celestial beings that are standing by to make our lives easier in all ways. Extending and reaching our arms toward the sky, we surrender in prayer.

It is preferable to cultivate faith and devotion *before* we are in desperate need. Wholehearted devotion connects us through faith to our source. Learning to trust the power within, we courageously let go and live each moment to the fullest. That, after all, is how life is doled out to us, one moment at a time. We then become intoxicated with the Divine.

> "Come to the edge, he said. They said, we are afraid. Come to the
> edge, he said. They came. He pushed them. And they flew!"
>
> —Guillaume Apolkinaire

Through wholehearted dedication (Iswara Pranidhana), *we become intoxicated with the Divine*.

EXPERIENCING THE POWER OF WHOLEHEARTED DEDICATED (*ISWARA PRANIDHANA*) PRAYER

Notice the times when you feel the desire to pray. Is it at times of joy, or times of unhappiness? If your prayers are always petitions, try re-forming them to express gratitude.

If you use praise, feeling you will receive something in return, affirm that blessings are abundant.

Begin to formulate an affirmation or prayer in your own words that allows you to expand into the next level of joy.

Repeat this prayer or affirmation at first in "formal" times in the morning and evening. Then begin to repeat it as many times during the day as possible, encouraging the repetition in both your mind and heart.

To help you to remember this gem during the day, place a colored dot on your watch, or a note on the computer, the telephone, the car ignition, or any place you frequent. Let it be a constant reminder, as you glance at it, to remember and repeat the affirmation or prayer.

In a week's time, change the wording to reflect yet another layer of your Divinity. Continue to grow and blossom as the joy comes forth.

HATHA YOGA:
Harmonizing Body, Breath, and Senses

W E NOW EXPERIENCE how the outward harmony of body, breath, and senses reveals our inner nature.

The natural comfort and joy of our being is expressed when the body becomes steady (asana).

As the body yields all efforts and holdings, the infinite within is revealed.

Thereafter we are freed from the fluctuations of the gunas.

The universal life force (prana) is enhanced and guided through the harmonious rhythm of the breath (pranayama).

The movement of the life force is influenced by inhalation, exhalation, and sustained breath.

A balanced, rhythmical pattern steadies the mind and emotions, causing the breath to become motionless.

As a result, the veils over the inner light are lifted.

The vista of higher consciousness is revealed.

Encouraging the senses to draw inward is pratyahara.

Glimpsing the inner light, the senses contentedly dwell within.

11.46 *The natural comfort and joy of our being is expressed when the body becomes steady (asana).*

11.47 *As the body yields all efforts and holdings, the infinite within is revealed.*

11.48 *Thereafter we are freed from the fluctuations of the* gunas.

The *Yama* and *Niyama* enable us to model the attitudes of Golden Age consciousness. We now venture to the next three facets of *Asthaanga Yoga,* known as *Hatha Yoga.* Their positioning after *Yama* and *Niyama* suggests that embracing a high level of behavior before beginning asana practice protects us from misusing or wasting the very powerful energy that is released. When we are firmly grounded in these principles, any unseemly thoughts or emotions are neither exacerbated nor strengthened.

HA-THA—A BALANCE OF ENERGIES

The complete system of *Hatha Yoga* increases vital energy by aligning our physical and subtle bodies, through physical poses (asana), guiding and enhancing the life force through breathing practices (*pranayama*), and encouraging the senses inward through deep relaxation (*pratyahara*). All three aspects were designed to be practiced in concert, thereby harmonizing body, breath, and senses.

When popularized in the West, the physical postures were isolated, excluding the other two aspects of *Hatha Yoga* almost completely. This oversight can encourage imbalances and injuries to the body, as well as to the mental and emotional well-being. Today most people commonly refer to the isolated practice of asana as the total system, simply calling it Yoga.

Ha-tha represents the integrated energy that then polarizes within each of us as light and dark, sun and moon, masculine and feminine. *Ha* represents the sun, heating, and "masculine" qualities of reason and intellectual thinking, while *tha* characterizes the moon, cooling, and "feminine" qualities of emotional and intuitive feelings. Each one of us has both the male *ha* and the female *tha* within us in varied proportions. The finer the balance, the more harmonious we feel.

When describing "asana," Sutra II. 46 uses two Sanskrit words: *sthira* and *sukha.*

Sthira denotes an effortlessness while coming into the pose or posture, holding it, or coming out of it.

Sukha reflects the natural state of comfort and joy. As the body finds its ease, the mind and emotions align with it, reflecting the light of the Divine. It allows us the feeling of being comfortable in our own skin. The inner and outer worlds interconnect.

The placement of the sutras on *Hatha Yoga* suggests they are a preparation for sitting meditation. Aching bodies distracted the ancient yogis in their quest to sit still. Unable to dedicate their focus inward, they realized that settling the mind was unlikely if even the slightest distraction remained in the body.

By practicing a few simple poses *before* sitting, you encourage a sense of comfort and ease in the body, the mind calms, and the spirit is more readily accessed. After all, a certain amount of discipline and physical strength is needed to keep the body in a steady seated position without movement for a half-hour or longer. Through asana practice, distractions of the body become infrequent visitors. The result is that we feel better, look better, and can project that feeling into our daily life.

The practice of asana encourages the body, mind, and breath to function together. The mind first decides on the movement and then directs the energy. The physical body, given the blueprint, follows. Much of our pain, stiffness, and disease is caused by the low quantity or impeded flow of energy in the body and mind.

Rhythmical breathing coordinated with this movement releases blockages and allows energy to flow. Holding the breath gives our nervous system a distress signal that is then sent to the organs, glands, and the muscular system. When it is flowing normally and rhythmically, the breath distributes energy through pathways, which encourage relaxation and the ability to stretch further.

Along with bringing ease to the body, the practice of asana was intended by the *sadhus* (spiritual seekers) to prepare their bodies for the intense physical rigor that was a fact of their lives. It was a very different time and culture from ours. When the practice of asana traversed the world, the need to adapt the poses for Western bodies became apparent. For example, from childhood to old age in most Asian countries, people commonly sit in a simple cross-legged pose. For them it is quite comfortable. If we at age thirty, forty, or fifty try to adapt that same simple pose, our knees may complain for days or longer afterward. When the adaptations are not heeded, we find the asanas difficult to do well and often, and the benefits will be overshadowed by frustration or injury.

THE FEMININE UNIQUENESS

It is also an important distinction to note that the asanas were designed for the needs of a male body. A woman's body and her emotional makeup have unique qualities that need special attention. Many of the poses need to be adapted to the female body. Yet our special needs are ignored if we follow traditional asana instruction rather than our intuition. While gentle pressure and squeezing help to improve blood circulation and health, too-vigorous bending and stretching can harm the softer and less muscular female body.

I would always joke with my students when teaching the *Mayurasana,* or Peacock, pose. In this pose, the entire weight of the body is balanced on bent arms as the elbows push into the belly so the straightened legs can be raised into the air. In order to accomplish this pose, the balance point must be at the center of the body (the elbows being the fulcrum). But the female pelvis is bigger and heavier than a man's, making the center of gravity lower. So if, adhering to the traditional instructions, the elbows are pushed into the abdomen, most women would fall forward and flat on their faces when they raised their legs. By pushing the elbows into the pelvis rather than the abdomen, we are more easily able to balance. However, while the elbows against the pelvis enable us to do the pose, they can put too much pressure on the delicate organs housed there. Injury or imbalance can occur. Since the position mimics a peacock (male) with long tail feathers splayed, I suggest women do a version I call *Peahen* pose, in which the legs are folded and tucked underneath the belly. In this way, the center of gravity shifts and the pose is accomplished.

The mental, emotional, and energetic aspects of asana can be as great if not greater than the physical aspect. When the mind images the benefits of a pose, the energy moves more easily to that part. Then we receive maximum benefits from the practice—a relaxed, healthy body and mind. All this stretching leads us to a supple body of health and strength that is able to be active, as well as to sit perfectly still.

On an emotional level, a woman's sensitivity often shifts to more of a masculine *Ha* if she continually takes on challenges and engages in competition. Instead of experiencing feelings of compassion when confronted with a situation, we may first exhibit anger. Because of the emphasis placed on our more masculine side, our feminine qualities are depleted instead of enhanced. Both aspects need to be honored.

Today there are hundreds of methods and schools for practicing Yoga poses. Choose the type of asana you want to practice, based not just on the physical benefits but also on how it will affect your emotional makeup. It is essential to understand what type of practice your particular temperament requires. Also, be aware of the effect that the practice is having on the subtle nervous system. If your nervous system is sensitive and you adapt a vigorous asana practice, it may cause an imbalance. Allow asana to be one part of your complete *Hatha Yoga* practice.

As the practice is established, it affords flexibility of body, mind, and emotions. With this comes balance and the yearning to be still and know yourself.

"The body itself is to reveal the light that's blazing inside your Presence."

—*Rumi*

The natural comfort and joy of our being is expressed when the body becomes steady (asana).

As the body yields all efforts and holdings, the infinite within is revealed.

Thereafter we are freed from the fluctuations of the gunas.

EXPERIENCING HOW THE THOUGHT INFLUENCES THE FLEXIBILITY OF THE BODY

Choose two asanas that you are familiar with, one that you can do with ease and love, and one that is a little more challenging for your body.

Begin to practice the one you love and notice why you like it. Is it because you are proficient at it or does it just feel good? Notice how the mind and the feelings react after you have finished.

Invoke the same happy feeling that came to you during the asana you love. Hold that feeling and transpose it on the other asana. If the mind starts to move into "I cannot do this well, I really do not like the way this one makes me feel," then bring the mind back to the happy feeling.

Soon you may experience a release replaced by a feeling of comfort and ease of the body that just a few moments before had seemed impossible.

II.49 *The universal life force* (prana) *is enhanced and guided through the harmonious rhythm of the breath* (pranayama).

II.50 *The movement of the life force is influenced through inhalation, exhalation, and sustained breath.*

Inhabiting and surrounding each cell of our physical body is the universal energy called *prana* (this energy is named *qi* in Japan and *chi* in China). Everything in the natural world has a field of energy surrounding and circulating through it. At different times the quality and quantity of *prana* may vary.

For example, a tree in winter would have less circulating *prana* than a tree in springtime. There is more energy needed for a tree to flower than to exist in the dormant stage. *Prana* is the intelligence that responds to the varying needs. *Prana* is similar to electricity in that it supplies an invisible current to keep life flowing and functioning.

At birth, we are allotted a quantity of this precious vital energy that continuously circulates, maintaining our function in daily life. Our first life-affirming action on this planet is to inhale, taking in the precious atmosphere of the earth, as well as a dose of *prana*. This action enlivens our bodies, making them suitable to sustain life in our new world. We then continue to breathe about sixteen times a minute, hopefully for many years to come. At a certain time, very near the last beat of our hearts, we return the borrowed air we took in at the beginning with an exhalation and go on our way, out of our body and to our next destination. In this way a breathing body is considered to be alive, and a breathless body is considered to be dead. What is often overlooked is that we are the indweller of the body, not the body itself.

While a substantial portion of *prana* is allotted for daily use, a greater amount is put "in trust" until the time comes to further our quest to know the Divine Self. A vast capacity of *prana* is needed to raise the energy from the physical to the spiritual realms. This "trust fund" is safely stored at the base of the spine, most often known as the Kundalini (coiled snake). Through the wide range of yogic practices, we slowly access this energy as it guides us to deeper levels of consciousness.

Our senses augment the already-circulating *prana*: through the beauty, we see; the sounds, we hear; the touch, we receive; the fragrance, we smell; the food, we eat. The sun, the moon, the stars, thoughts, emotions, actions, and words all have the capacity to enhance or diminish our *prana*.

THE SUBTLE NERVOUS SYSTEM

It is estimated that there are between 150,000 and 300,000 subtle pathways, or *nadis*, within and surrounding the physical body. The purpose of these *nadis* is to circulate and distribute the much-needed energy to the physical, mental, and emotional bodies (*koshas*). The *nadis* function in a similar way to the blood vessels. Of the many thousand of *nadis*, three are most significant: *Ida, Pingala,* and *Shushumna.*

The *Pingala Nadi* and *Ida Nadi* polarize the neutral energy as they wind around the spinal cord. The *prana* circulates through the *Pingala Nadi* (the *ha,* or sun in *Hatha*), generating heat and the masculine attributes of rational thinking and intellectual reasoning. The *Pingala* governs the sympathetic nervous system and corresponds to the left side of the brain.

When *prana* circulates through the *Ida Nadi* (the *THA,* or moon in *Hatha*), it produces a coolness and accesses the feminine attributes of emotion, feelings, and intuition. *Ida* guides the parasympathetic nervous system and corresponds with the right side of the brain.

The *Shushumna Nadi* only comes into play when the *Pingala* and *Ida* are in perfect harmony. It then has the sacred duty to carry the *prana* through to the higher centers of consciousness (chakras). It does not function as the day-to-day distributor of energy to the physical, mental, or emotional bodies.

The universal life force (prana) *is enhanced and guided through the harmonious rhythm of the breath* (pranayama).

The movement of the life force is influenced by inhalation, exhalation, and sustained breath.

This refined circulation of *prana* is possible because of our sophisticated system of breathing, which facilitates this process much as the pumping heart does for the circulatory system. Through the steady rhythm of inhalation *(Puraka)* and exhalation *(Rechaka)*, the air and *prana* circulate within and between the physical and subtle bodies. The inhalation draws the *prana* to the center of our being, and with the exhalation it journeys outward. All this happens within the breath's regular pattern of sixteen times a minute. A slight hesitation *(Kumbaka)* between the inhalation and the exhalation allows oxygen as well as the precious *prana* to be distributed.

THE CHANGING PATTERNS

Having two nostrils supports the flow of energy through *Pingala* and *Ida*. Although most of us are probably unaware of it, the lining of each nostril engorges and shrinks periodically during the day. This shifts the flow of air from one nostril to the other in a biological rhythm. Every one and a half to three hours the *Pingala* and the *Ida* alternate dominance, in hopes of restoring balance. Extreme heat or cold can also cause the nostrils to change or switch dominance. Allowing the air to pass through the right or left nostril produces a heating or cooling effect, respectively. Outside on a cold winter's day—even though you are not aware of it—your right nostril is fully open and desperately trying to heat the body. When the environment suddenly changes as you walk into an overheated room, your right nostril will occlude, and the left will go on duty. This alternating pattern becomes more obvious when you have a head cold that stuffs up your nose. Usually one of the nostrils opens just enough to let some airflow through. When both nostrils are completely clogged, we resort to using the only viable alternative, the mouth, to breathe.

All of our physical systems depend on the regular flow of air *and* of *prana*. If our habitual breathing patterns are upset or halted because of erratic movements in our body, the oxygen and energy requirements go up. If we suddenly run or quicken our pace, the breath accelerates, using up more *prana*. As we slow down, our breath follows.

If our bodies can change our breathing pattern, then the opposite is also true. A deep breath revitalizes us when we are tired. When we observe how these variations in breathing change our breathing according to our daily functions and moods, *pranayama* becomes an essential practice in returning us to balance.

Mental states affect the breathing pattern and also change nostril dominance. When we feel anger *or* passion, which are heating emotions, chances are our right nostril will be open. Depression or a sense of quietness may cause the left nostril to take over. At night, as the nostril dominance shifts, we turn from one side to the other. Whichever side we are lying on, the opposite nostril is open. If you nap in the heat of day, the left nostril's vigilance allows you to rest deeply. If, suddenly, the phone rings, disturbing your sleep, the left nostril will engorge, causing the right nostril to release and allowing you to be present for the call. The body's consciousness is awake even when we are sleeping.

The mind and emotions host millions of thoughts and feelings that are perpetually hungry for energy in order to move about and function. These thoughts and feelings respond to the same rhythmical relationship the breath has with the body. With a long, slow exhalation, they have room to spread out. The measured, rhythmical pace allows them time to consider whether and how they will manifest. This is similar to the spacing of notes in music. The greater the spacing between the notes, the more relaxing effect the music produces. Awareness of the breath can boost the enjoyment and vitality of each moment of life.

When a balance between the *Pingala* and the *Ida* is sustained over a period of time through various *pranayama* practices, the *prana* is then directed through the central *nadi*, the *Shushumna*. This centers the mind and emotions, moving them toward the highest consciousness *(Samadhi)*.

The universal life force (prana) *is enhanced and guided through the harmonious rhythm of the breath* (pranayama).

The movement of the life force is influenced by inhalation, exhalation, and sustained breath.

MAGNETIZE YOURSELF TOWARD BALANCE AND HARMONY

Taking in a deep breath has the effect of "combing" our energy. When we visit the mirror after we wake up, we usually see that our hair is in disarray. We're unfazed, since we learned early on that a strategically placed comb or brush could coax the hairs to go more or less in the same direction. Satisfied, we look and feel a bit more in control (at least of our hair!). Breathing practices have the same effect on our energy field, our *pranic* body. With rhythmical breathing, we align and "comb" the energy; it becomes smoother, calmer, and more focused. This focused energy then acts like a magnet, attracting like polarities to us.

In a plain piece of metal, all the molecules are in chaos facing every which way. A magnet is a similar piece of metal in which all the molecules are perfectly aligned—the north poles facing one way, and the south poles facing in the opposite direction. Because of this alignment, the magnet gains the power to attract and hold other objects. If you stroke the ordinary metal and the magnet together in one direction only, the magnet will align all the molecules in the plain metal with itself, causing a second magnet to emerge. The power to attract and hold has been transmitted from one to the other, while amazingly enough the initial magnet retains its full strength. If you now take the two magnets and stroke them so the repelling poles are facing each other, the strength of each will diminish. The power to attract and hold is gone. We can see the benefit of being with those that support us rather than neutralize our power (*satsang*).

The universal life force (prana) *is enhanced and guided through the harmonious rhythm of the breath* (pranayama).

The movement of the life force is influenced by inhalation, exhalation, and sustained breath.

As we align our energies in this way, through regulating the breath, we maintain calm through the ordinary emotional rollercoaster rides we encounter each day. We find that when we are upset, everything around us reflects the same disturbance, as if it is somehow contagious. When tranquillity prevails, it magnetizes everything with the same sense of calmness.

BREATH, MIND, AND EMOTIONS IN HARMONY

Children allow us to see how our thoughts and emotions are linked with the breath. When they become frightened, their breath and speech patterns change. Often they will come running in breathlessly to tell us of some disturbing event that happened. The breath, trying to form words, tells us the child is upset: "Mo . . . Mommy! Hahuha (hic) ahhh hahu (sob)!!!"

"Sweetie, I can see you are very upset, but I can't understand what you're saying. Please calm down and tell me what happened."

Meanwhile, *your* breath has become irregular as visions of a horrible incident fill your wild imagination. You want to be able to calm your child, but how? Embracing her, you softly kiss her forehead, and say, "Sweetie, take a deep breath. Now let it out slowly. Again. Good. Now, can you tell me what happened?" Her words can now be understood because her breath is in harmony with her thoughts and emotions. Fortunately, the crisis was not as monumental as you had imagined it to be. (It rarely is!)

What you were witnessing and experiencing was the child's breath mimicking the pattern of her thoughts and emotions. The mind picks up the erratic flow of breath and begins to get more excited, unaware that the mind itself was the cause of this irregularity. This then causes the breath to become more erratic, thus causing a cycle that is difficult to interrupt. The child was trying to tell you what happened, but she couldn't because her breath, guided by the mind and emotions, was too disturbed.

The traumas of childhood have become everyday occurrences in adulthood. Our thoughts and emotions may be just as chaotic and upset, but we have learned ways to keep the stressful thoughts and feelings trapped inside, and, from that, a greater disharmony manifests.

Next time you find yourself agitated with daily irritants, notice your breath. Chances are you are taking in a breath, holding it, and then letting it out quickly. Take a moment and adjust the pattern—have your breath flow in and out without hesitation or strain. The more upset you are, the more difficult this will seem. Stay with it for a minute or longer, and you will be amazed how the thoughts and feelings respond.

The universal life force (prana) *is enhanced and guided through the harmonious rhythm of the breath* (pranayama).

The movement of the life force is influenced by inhalation, exhalation, and sustained breath.

11.51 *A balanced, rhythmical pattern steadies the mind and emotions, causing the breath to become motionless.*

11.52 *As a result, the veils over the inner light are lifted.*

11.53 *The vista of higher consciousness is revealed.*

Pranayama's physical and mental effects have the supreme purpose of leading us into the stillness necessary for meditation. It is a wonderful practice to be done immediately before meditation. Asana steadies the body; *pranayama* aligns the mental and emotional patterns. We will then guide the senses through *pratyahara*, allowing us to focus and dive deep within.

Through the continual practice of *pranayama*, the breath will understand that its workload has been greatly reduced. As the inhalation and exhalation slow, their stillness initiates the phase of motionless breath. It is a very natural and comfortable state, unlike the strained holding of breath we witness when upset. With a deepening in meditation, the *prana*, mind, and emotions grow still, causing a spontaneous stoppage of the breath (*Kevala Kumbaka*). The *prana* moves inward, flowing through the *Shushumna* to merge with the energy stored in the spine (Kundalini), which then moves magnetically upward, propelling us to higher consciousness.

The practice of *pranayama* slowly allows the veils covering our true self to lift. We are able to ascend unencumbered toward the light and merge with our Divine nature.

A balanced, rhythmical pattern steadies the mind and emotions, causing the breath to become motionless.

As a result, the veils over the inner light are lifted.

The vista of higher consciousness is revealed.

EXPERIENCING A BALANCE OF THE *PINGALA* (MASCULINE) AND THE *IDA* (FEMININE) THROUGH ALTERNATE-NOSTRIL BREATHING

(Please note: This breathing practice allows us to utilize the full lung capacity, taking in approximately seven times the amount of oxygen as in our normal shallow breathing. The chest muscles and the lungs may not be accustomed to such expansion, so be extra alert to any strain or dizziness. If you begin to get tired or short of breath, return to normal breathing for a few breaths; and then, after resting, continue. This will help to build up your stamina without strain. Strain or stress actually depletes the life force, erasing many of the good effects from the breathing practice.)

This breathing practice is done in a comfortable seated position. It is a great practice to do anytime to calm yourself, or as a wonderful gateway to meditation.

With the right hand, make a gentle fist and release the thumb, the ring finger, and the little finger. This is a classic hand position in Yoga, called Vishnu Mudra (Sustaining Seal). If it is uncomfortable, you can use the thumb and index finger. The thumb gently presses the right nostril closed while the left nostril remains open. Then, the extended fingers gently close the left nostril and the thumb releases the right nostril. (The left hand is resting comfortably on the lap.)

To begin, exhale fully through both nostrils. Close off the right nostril with your thumb and inhale slowly through the left nostril as you expand the belly and the lower lungs. Continue to inhale to the upper chest. Feel the collarbones rise slightly.

Close off the left nostril with the fingers and exhale through the right nostril, releasing the air from the upper chest, the lower chest, and the abdomen—one section flowing into the other.

Inhale through the right nostril, expanding the abdomen and lower chest, the middle chest, and the upper chest, so that the collarbones rise slightly. Close off the right nostril with the thumb and exhale through the left nostril.

Continue this pattern. Exhale, inhale, switch nostrils; exhale, inhale, switch. Begin to practice for one minute and gradually increase up to three minutes or longer.

At the end of three minutes, as you come around to the right nostril, end with an exhalation. Allow the hand to come to the lap. Be still for a few moments with the eyes closed as you observe how calm and still the breath and mind have become. Observe the relationship between the two.

II.54 *Encouraging the senses to draw inward is* pratya-hara.

II.55 *Glimpsing the inner light, the senses contentedly dwell within.*

Pratyahara is the subtlest aspect of *Hatha Yoga*. It is a prelude to meditation. Most meditation techniques begin by enticing the senses to draw inward, allowing the mind to follow.

The five sense (*manas*), encouraged by curiosity (*ahamkara*), link up with the intellect (*buddhi*) and coax us outward from our inner consciousness. Even before birth, the senses feed us enormous amounts of information for both survival and enjoyment. With time, if we engage exclusively in the outer sphere of the senses, our inner world is forgotten.

Incredibly powerful, our senses expose us to the infinite spectrum of the universe. For thousands of years we have been awed and humbled by the sun, the moon, and the night sky. By developing highly refined instruments, we observe the far reaches of the universe, which are merely the portals to the multitude of undiscovered worlds millions of light-years away.

Venturing outward into the cosmic universe has triggered a polarity that draws us deeper within, creating a passion for the miraculous workings of the human body. Traveling inward with the help of technology, we explore atoms, DNA strands, and subatomic particles that we have yet to meet. Persistent in investigating both frontiers, we hope to learn the secrets to our existence.

With spiritual maturity, our inward explorations go beyond the physical world to explore the mystical fields. This necessitates a relaxation on the grasp our outer senses have on the external world. Because of the degree of overstimulation (*Rajas*) in our modern society, this can be a difficult shift. Accustomed to going every which way they please, the senses need to be cajoled as they rotate inward toward this new journey. If this overstimulation prevails on the inward focus, it stirs agitation and disharmony in our mind and emotions. This is why at the onset of inward practice, some report that they feel *less peaceful* than before. But with continuous guidance from the *Yamas* and *Niyamas,* the senses grow calm.

Encouraging the senses to draw inward is pratyahara.

Glimpsing the inner light, the senses contentedly dwell within.

THE BEAUTY OF THE SUBTLE WORLDS
DRAWS US INWARD

Gently enticing the senses to draw within often starts with our strongest information-gatherer: the power of sight. More than 75 percent of information gathered from the external world is assembled from what we *see*.

Redirecting the seeing to an internal focus encourages all the other senses to follow. Because we load so many visual images in our minds, we continue to "see" even with the eyes closed. Often students learning to meditate are coached to establish their inward gaze between the eyebrows (to their "third eye") or at the heart center. With this slow and gentle training, the mind will gradually relinquish its projection of previously imprinted visual images.

Carefully choosing our outward images can help the inner vision to calm. Watching a visually frightening movie encourages the reflection of the same forces in our innermost worlds. At times it might be difficult to know if the images have staked a temporary or permanent residency within your mind. For a deeper level of practice, you may choose to withdraw, even temporarily, to a simple place in nature that affords very little outward stimulation.

As the "sight" firmly adheres to the inner world, the sense of hearing follows. Refining the level and quality of sound we regularly experience prepares us for the subtle internal sounds. The innermost melodies are orchestrated by the *prana* as it travels through the subtle nerve channels *(nadis)*. We become captivated by a delicate hum or swish as it transforms into the celestial sound of bells, whispers, and choirs of angels.

DEVELOPING EXTRA-ORDINARY SENSES

The subtler senses of touch, smell, and taste join seeing and hearing in their quest for inner vistas. As the senses find comfort in their inward journey, the "ordinary" senses become refined and powerful. We have tapped into the subtle realm of "extrasensory perception." What we then "see" is not physical. We "hear" what has not yet been said, "smell" what is not apparent, "feel" what we know to be true. These are some of the extraordinary powers described in the *Yoga Sutras* in Book III, *"Vibhuti Pada:* The Divine Manifestation of Power," as the fruits of spiritual practice.

A mother can often "see" what her child is doing even if the child is out of "normal sight." Sometimes mothers are said to have eyes in the back of their heads because they "see" beyond the normal scope of vision.

Moments before her death, Saint Thérèse of Lisieux, known as the Little Flower, saw a vision of Mother Mary surrounded by hundreds of roses. Although those present in the room could not *see* this vision, the overwhelming fragrance of roses permeated the room. From that day forward, anyone who prayed to Saint Thérèse knew their prayers were heard when the unmistakable *scent of roses* enveloped the room.

Encouraging the senses to draw inward is pratyahara.

Glimpsing the inner light, the senses contentedly dwell within.

Often we learn of situations in which someone was warned of impending danger by a voice not connected to a physical body.

I experienced such a lifesaving voice while camping by a lazy river in the Colorado Mountains. Having pitched the tent and eaten to our appetites' fill, it was time to snuggle into our sleeping bags and be lulled to sleep by the sounds of nature. A river's voice can be the perfect lullaby.

Not remembering drifting off to sleep, I was suddenly and quite rudely awakened by a voice. Loud and clear it said, "Get up right now, pull up your tent, collect all your gear, and head for higher ground."

I peeked outside, and the moon's reflection on the water told my "regular" senses that everything was as it should be. But why did this voice wake me with such a message? Trusting that I was given this warning for a reason, I timidly woke my tentmate.

More than a bit annoyed, she acquiesced to my emphatic rendition of the "higher" communication that I heard. We pulled up camp and spent the rest of the night restlessly sleeping in our car in front of a restaurant that was closed for the night.

The next morning dawned clear and bright, and I was ready to concede defeat, accepting all the teasing I surely deserved. Eating breakfast in the restaurant, we overheard the other patrons talking with great concern about how last night the river rose and flooded out the banks. "Sure hope no one was camping there," I heard several people say, as I said silent prayers of gratitude—not only that I was warned, but that I had listened!

Once asked by a keen student how she could develop her extrasensory perception, Sri Swami Satchidanandaji smiled and said, "Why would you want to take on *extra* when you have difficulty handling the ordinary senses you have now? If you invite these extrapowerful senses, make sure you are strong enough to handle them."

The external world will fail to amuse the senses as you create an extraordinary world within. Entice the senses inward by invoking a gentle light or flame, the sound of your heartbeat, the fragrance of roses, the sweetness of saliva, or a feeling of well-being. Find ways to see, hear, and feel beauty in the delicate world within. As the outward senses are calm, meditation becomes effortless.

Encouraging the senses to draw inward is pratyahara.

Glimpsing the inner light, the senses contentedly dwell within.

EXPERIENCING THE SENSES AND AWARENESS DRAWING INWARD

This is a profound relaxation practice for bringing in all of the outward sensual consciousness. We begin with the physical body, then move to the breath, thoughts, and emotions.

Begin to take in a few deep breaths. Notice how still the body and breath become as they relax. Observe the breath without controlling it as it comes and goes without any strain.

Guide this gentle breath to bring all sensual awareness from the feet, ankles, lower legs, knees, thighs, hips. Relax.

Guide this awareness to withdraw from the fingers, hands, wrists, forearms, elbows, upper arms.

Let go of holding awareness in the hands and arms, or shoulders. Relax.

Do the same with the buttocks and pelvis, allow the abdomen to soften, imagine the chest, lungs, the heart, and the throat relaxed.

Gently allow the awareness from the base of the spine to slowly rise up through the middle spine to the upper spine. Relax the shoulders and allow the neck to be an open connection between the heart and the head. Relax.

Experience the sensations as the body retreats.

The head holds most of the organs of the senses. Gently relax the jaw and withdraw taste and speech from the mouth.

Withdraw smell from the nose.

Allow the eyelids and the eyes to soften, moving toward the inner sight.

Relax the forehead, and tune the ears to the inner sounds. Relax the entire scalp and bathe the brain with relaxation.

Allow the gentle breath to relieve the mind and emotions of all movement. Relax.

Slowly bring the awareness to the gentle breath as it enters and leaves the body.

As it enters, feel yourself drawing deeper within.

As it leaves, feel yourself letting go of all holdings.

Notice a lightness and a feeling of distancing from the body, mind, emotions, and all worldly cares.

Begin to go further within to look for that place of stillness, peace, and joy. This is the dwelling place of your Divine Self.

(Have five full minutes of quiet time.)

Slowly and gently bring the awareness back to the breath.

Begin to increase the inhalation and feel that the senses have been purified and strengthened. Begin to feel them awakening to a relaxed body and a calm mind.

As you continue with this practice, your senses will become accustomed to drawing inward. It will become effortless to prepare the mind and emotions for deeper practice.

BOOK III.

VIBHUTI PADA:

The Divine Manifestation of Power

Book III begins with the last three sutras of the Eight-Faceted Path
(Asthaanga Yoga): Dharana *(contemplation),* Dhyana *(meditation),*
and Samadhi *(Union with Divine Consciousness). These final three*
facets are more internal than the preceding five, and as they flow
seamlessly from one to another, they are known as Samyama
(fusion). With Samyama *comes perfect knowledge of the Divine*
Self. Accompanying this realization is the manifestation (Vibhuti) of
psychic and spiritual powers (siddhis). The culmination of Book III
describes the myriad powers born of the fusion (Samyama) of
Dharana, Dhyana, *and* Samadhi.

Please note: I have chosen to present commentary on only the first
five sutras in Book III, "Vibhuti Pada: The Divine Manifestation of
Power." The remaining sutras of Book III, and all of Book IV,
"Kaivalya Pada: Supreme Liberation," will be summarized in lieu of

*an explanation of the individual sutras. Books III and IV portray the
most esoteric aspects of the sutras, and they tend to be less useful for
creating the foundation of our spiritual quest.*

*Also, because of their esoteric nature, a heart-centered perspective
would not necessarily enhance the interpretation of these sutras in
the same way it did for Books I and II. As your curiosity about Books
III and IV develops, I encourage you to read the many translations
available.*

ANTARA YOGA:
The Inner Quest

WHEN THE FIVE preceding facets of *Asthaanga* have been effectively interwoven, we are gifted by *Antara Yoga*, the Inner Quest. With continued devotion, *Dharana* (contemplation) and *Dhyana* (meditation) guide us to the innermost treasure, *Samadhi* (Union with Divine Consciousness). When they seamlessly flow from one to another, it is known as *Samyama* (fusion).

> *Gathering consciousness and focusing it within is*
> Dharana (*contemplation*).

> *The continuous inward flow of consciousness is*
> Dhyana (*meditation*).

> *When individual consciousness unites with the*
> *Divine Consciousness, the illusion of separateness*
> *dissolves; this is* Samadhi.

> *When* Dharana (*contemplation*), Dhyana (*meditation*),
> *and* Samadhi (*Union with Divine Consciousness*)
> *seamlessly merge into one another, this is*
> Samyama (*fusion*).

> *Through* Samyama, *individual and Divine*
> *Consciousness gracefully reunite.*

III.1 *Gathering consciousness and focusing it within is* Dharana *(contemplation).*

It always intrigues me that *only* five of the eight facets of *Asthaanga Yoga* have commentaries in Book II, "*Sadhana Pada:* Cultivation of Spiritual Practice." The last three, *Dharana* (contemplation), *Dhyana* (meditation), and *Samadhi* (Union with Divine Consciousness), are designated to Book III, "*Vibhuti Pada*." It affirms that they are not practices in themselves; rather, they are progressive internal states that evolve from the earlier cultivated practices. Opening the doors to the Divine Manifestation of Power, "doing" transforms into "being."

If we are well primed, the transition to these subtle levels from the other preceding practices is effortless. Many may choose to "do meditation," but this is more often than not a technique derived from *pratyahara* practice (encouraging the senses inward).

Following the flow of *Yamas* and *Niyamas* as the first two facets of *Asthaanga Yoga,* we know that, as we develop reverence and devotion for others and ourselves, the mind and emotions become tranquil. Asana and *pranayama,* the third and fourth facets, allow the life force to gather and refine, bringing ease to the body, mind, and emotions. Then, *pratyahara,* the fifth facet, encourages the senses inward. Each of the facets, when practiced with dedication and respect, naturally leads us to the threshold of the Divine Manifestation of Power. It is a progression that can be neither quickened nor affected.

Observing the potential beauty of a rosebud, we may be eager to see it in full bloom. Becoming impatient with the process and taking nature into our own hands, if we peel the petals, hoping to create a full bloom, it would destroy both the sweet bud and the exquisite blossom. Maturity cannot be forced; it takes time, patience, and nurturing. Nature is a great teacher, showing us that everything develops at the perfect time.

The three graduated stages that are presented in these sutras are meant to exhibit a quantitative rather than qualitative difference. The same attention and awareness that is present in *Dharana* (contemplation) is also brought to *Dhyana* (meditation) and the lower states of *Samadhi* (Union with Divine Consciousness). The different phases are determined by the length of time our consciousness is able to remain engaged within.

Imagine this process similar to applying oil to a tough piece of leather, so that it may become supple. The length of time the oil is allowed to remain on the leather is crucial to the process. For it to soak in and soften the leather, it is best to leave it on for a long time. If the oil is applied and then removed within twenty seconds, the softening effect is minimal. If it stays for two minutes, the absorption process is able to begin. When the oil remains on the leather for half an hour or longer, it is completely absorbed, leaving the leather pliable and without a residue.

This is similar to the way *Dharana* (contemplation), *Dhyana* (meditation), and *Samadhi* (Union with Divine Consciousness) respectively affect the realization of our Divine Self. As we are able to gather our awareness and engage it within for a short amount of time, we are experiencing *Dharana*. If engaged for a longer time, we experience *Dhyana*. Yet more time allows for total absorption, *Samadhi*.

AN EASEFUL AWARENESS

Dharana is most commonly translated as "concentration" and is frequently used synonymously and interchangeably with the word "meditation." Defining it as "concentration" suggests an intense focusing of the mind. This characterization can cause our bodies to tense and our breathing to become irregular, and while our senses are alerted to the mission at hand, there is little comfort or ease. More accurately, *Dharana* invites us into an easeful awareness that prompts the flow of consciousness to return back to its source. In choosing an English equivalent for *Dharana,* "contemplation" or "reflection" is more in keeping with the effect we want to evoke.

Through *Dharana,* our thoughts, feelings, and actions interweave, inducing a pattern of consciousness that flows harmoniously to the source.

Gathering consciousness and focusing it within is Dharana (contemplation).

HARMONIZE WITH YOUR TRUE VIBRATION

In Book I, Sutras 34–38, we are offered a selection of uplifting ways to lead the mind and emotions to *Dharana* and *Dhyana.* The sutras, being very empowering and nonrestrictive, after offering us many choices, ultimately leave the path open ended. For example, I. 39: *Or dedicate yourself to anything that elevates and embraces your heart.* These two simple criteria for selecting a focus, elevation and embracing, seem agreeable to most anyone.

The first part of Sutra I. 39 suggests that the focus be both uplifting *and* inspiring. This gives you the freedom to choose almost anything you wish: a chakra or a spiritual center on the body, a great and inspiring being, a prayer or a sacred word; the options are infinite. Choose carefully, so that the qualities held within the sacred object will have the power to escort you to the depth of your Divine Self.

The second suggestion is that you love it, and that it elevates you to a state of joy. When you select something you love, your heart will want to embrace it fully.

Many of us have experienced elevating feelings from being in love. At those times our complete awareness is funneled into one special person—all of our senses and thoughts are with them; just to think about them uplifts us and brings joy.

Imagine you're at an airport waiting for your sweetheart. While standing there, waiting for the aircraft to come in, your feet may hurt a bit, or hunger may remind you that in your haste, you forgot to eat. But, the moment you see your beloved, energy suddenly floods your body, leaping out through your heart and rushing to embrace her or him. Your aching feet and hunger are long forgotten.

The experience of contemplation is usually not quite as visceral or dramatic. Yet, if we truly love what we are focusing on, with time and practice, the energy flows to the centers of higher consciousness, propelled by our devotion. We are filled with joy and bliss.

Even if you are given a focus for practice by a teacher, or learn one from a tried-and-true tradition, it is important to adapt it as you embrace it with your whole heart.

A friend of mine, who had a longtime career as a cardiac surgeon, went on a ten-day meditation retreat. When he returned, I asked him how the experience had been for him. "Oh, it was fine," he answered, still somewhat preoccupied. "Tell me something," he said. "They told us to meditate on the 'hara' [an energy center used in the Buddhist tradition]. I spent the whole time trying to figure out exactly where it was. Dusting off my memory, I went through my old *Gray's Anatomy* book from medical school, but I couldn't find the *hara*. I kept wondering if it was to the left or right, above or below the pancreas. Can you help clarify it for me?"

Chuckling to myself and at the same time appreciating his dilemma, I said, "Let's make this easy. Do you know where your heart is?"

"Of course I know where my heart is—and everybody else's, too," answered the experienced surgeon.

"Put your full and complete attention at the heart center and all the love that flows through it. That seems to be a perfect focus for you!" I said. He looked relieved as a smile appeared in his sparkling eyes.

In this case my friend was offered a focus that was not in harmony with his vibration. When you settle on something suited for you, become completely devoted to it. Sometimes after a while, we become impatient, thinking, "Oh, this technique is not working for me." We may then read a book or hear a teacher proclaim a "better way" and decide to try that approach. By switching techniques, you will not reach the depth or steadiness that you need to find your true center.

GO DEEP

There's a popular adage about digging shallow wells: If you dig down ten feet in one well and hit rock and then move to another place and dig down ten feet to no avail and then move again, you may never get water. But if you continue to dig deeply in one well—thirty, forty feet—eventually, you will be rewarded.

If you spend your energy continuously digging shallow wells, you will not know where to go to find refuge when something happens during the day to upset your equilibrium. Being faithful to one method, you can dive deep into that safe haven and merge with the inner stillness.

You may feel you are still "playing the field" with a variety of techniques. Gradually begin to embrace *one* closest to your temperament, and "date" only that one for a while. After a few weeks, you might get "engaged" to it, or you may decide it is not for you. Then select another. Stay with that one for a month or so. After two or three tries, choose *one,* make your "marriage" plans, and be faithful to your choice. Apply wholehearted devotion and let it escort you to your own heart, deep within.

Gathering consciousness and focusing it within is **Dharana** *(contemplation).*

EXPERIENCING CONTEMPLATION (*DHARANA*)
THROUGH *TRADAKA*, OR GAZING

(Please note: This practice is a wonderful example of *Pratya-hara* flowing into *Dharana*. It begins with an external physical focus and then draws you inward to the subtle image. It then alternates both an outward and inward focus, coordinating the eyes with the mind and emotions so they function as one. The outward gaze toward the external object is "seen" when we close our eyes by our inner vision. As the internal image dims, we again open our eyes and gaze outward to the physical form of the image. The practice is continued until our consciousness gathers and is persuaded to remain inward as *Dharana* (contemplation).

Choose an inspirational object: a lit candle, a photo, flowers, the sunrise or sunset, a mandala or yantra (which is a sacred geometric pattern), or anything that uplifts and evokes a quiet, peaceful feeling.

Sit directly in front of it so it is at eye level, close enough for you to see the form and feel its qualities.

(Because it is not necessary to distinguish details, glasses or contact lenses may be removed, permitting the eyes to relax and soften.)

Close your eyes. Take in a few deep breaths and let them out slowly as your body stills.

Slowly open the eyes halfway. Begin to gaze at your chosen object; the eyes and eyelids remain relaxed and soft.

Resist the temptation to reach out and grasp the image with your vision; instead, keep the eyes soft; allow the image to flow toward you.

At first, the eyes may wander. Gently bring them back to the chosen object. The breath continues to be gentle.

Allow the eyes to be directed outward until they blink, tear, or feel any discomfort. Then close them softly.

Observe the image as it now appears in the mind's eye. Gently perceive the same inspirational qualities as you go deep within.

When the inner image begins to fade, open the eyes again and gaze toward the external object.

If the mind starts to wander and brings in stories about the object, or something totally unrelated, gently bring your awareness back to the object in front of you.

Repeat this sequence several times, gazing outward and gazing inward.

Let all thoughts and feelings drift into the background as you contemplate your sacred object.

If any tension creeps into the body, take in a few deep breaths and let it go.

After a few minutes, allow the eyes to close, drawing deep within. Clearly "see" the image with the inner eye. Be silent for a few minutes and enjoy the inner stillness of Dharana.

III.2 *The continuous inward flow of consciousness is* Dhyana (*meditation*).

With continued inward awareness, *Dharana* (contemplation) transports us into *Dhyana* (meditation).

In *Dharana* (contemplation), the length of time consciousness dwells with the Divine is limited to a few seconds, causing the sense of peace we derive from *Dharana* to be transient. In *Dhyana* (meditation), the gathered consciousness nestles more comfortably into our Divine essence.

The distinction between the two stages is similar to the action of oil (awareness) being poured from a small vessel (*chitta*) back into the infinite sea (*chit*). *Dharana* intermittently touches inner awareness, similar to the way oil pours from a *full* cylinder, stopping ever so briefly before the next plop follows. There is a definite start and end to the periods of inner awareness, and often they happen so quickly that we miss the inner experience.

Because of these frequent fluctuations in the state of *Dharana,* our awareness vacillates from the external to the internal, between "doing" and "being," back and forth. *Dhyana* (meditation) is analogous to the oil (awareness), flowing in a *continuous* stream from the small vessel (*chitta*) back to the infinite (*chit*) sea of consciousness. With *Dhyana,* the awareness remains within for a longer time. This allows our identification with the Divine to increase. Even when the "formal" meditation is completed, a part of us is always rooted within.

Dhyana propels our consciousness toward the vast sea of the Divine. Less-determined thoughts and emotions are coaxed to flow with it toward the source. This dynamic experience of meditation brims over, touching every aspect of life. The aura (*pranic* body) becomes luminous with this dynamic power, giving you a magnetic and vibrant personality. As this power continues to deepen, people are drawn to you and are affected by your cheerfulness, your immeasurable energy, and your joy. Your peace and strength are elevated by the boundless source that you have accessed. The unpleasant situations that you once avoided are now understood, and in some cases welcomed. You are able to observe that all things have a greater purpose, even if that purpose is sometimes hidden. People you once experienced as foreign or strange can be embraced by your open and loving heart. A whole new perspective has unfolded.

The continuous inward flow of consciousness is Dhyana (meditation).

You may find it necessary to withdraw from the world for a time to continue nourishing this dynamic power. Or, as is often the case with this newfound energy, you may find yourself inspired to serve others and yourself with greater zeal.

The state of *Dhyana* expands our understanding of the world around us, and of ourselves. We are able to delight in the newfound bliss that up to this time had been held in reserve. In *Dhyana* we transcend the physical, mental, and emotional realms, and we experience infinite joy.

The continuous inward flow of consciousness is Dhyana (meditation).

EXPERIENCING THE MEDITATIVE STATE (*DHYANA*)

Sit in a comfortable position, relax the body and breath, and allow the senses to draw inward. Focus the awareness on the place between the eyebrows, the third eye.

As you become still, observe the sound of the breath as it enters the body and whispers the sound "So." Listen to the breath as it leaves. "Hum." "So-Hum. So-Hum."

Join the breath by silently repeating "So" with the inhalation. Silently repeat "Hum" with the exhalation. (This is japa, *repetition of a mantra.)*

"So-Hum," "So-Hum," "So-Hum." (This invokes the vibration of "I Am.")

Listen to the whisper of the rhythm of life as it flows in and out of the body. It is affirming both nature ("So") and spirit ("Hum"). Recognizing both parts of us in harmony, it calls us to the light within.

"So-Hum." "So-Hum." "So-Hum." "So-Hum." "So-Hum." "So-Hum." "So-Hum."

Continue listening as you softly repeat this mantra for ten minutes or longer.

After a time allow the "So-Hum" mantra to repeat itself (ajapa). *"So-Hum" will take you to the place where the body, mind, and breath dissolve into the Divine.*

III.3 *When individual consciousness unites with the Divine Conciousness, the illusion of separateness dissolves; this is* Samadhi.

The world that we visit during *Samadhi* (Union with Divine Consciousness) has no tangible language. It is a state beyond description. It can only be experienced.

If we stir a cup of sugar into a pitcher of water, it *seems* to disappear. We may not be able to *see* it, yet, if we *taste* the water, we recognize the sugar by its sweetness. Because the sugar has been completely absorbed in the water, their union creates a new expression. From then on it becomes impossible to separate the two.

The effect of the sugar merging with the water is similar to our gathered consciousness merging into the Divine. When consciousness unites in *Samadhi,* unlike *Dharana* (contemplation) or *Dhyana* (meditation), the distinction between the individual consciousness (*chitta*) and the eternal consciousness (*chit*) dissolves.

Trying to comprehend *Samadhi* (Union with Divine Consciousness) before we have experienced it is like trying to understand being in love before it happens. A child might ask her mother what it feels like to be "in love." With great introspection, her mother may answer, "It is not something that can be explained in words. It is beyond our understanding of what joy can mean. All I can say is you will know it when it happens!" *Samadhi* is like that.

The different stages and degrees of *Samadhi* (Union with Divine Consciousness) are described and defined in Book I, Chapter 7, Sutras 40–51. As we might remember, some of these elevated states are temporary (*Sabija*); they still hold seeds that can sprout. These states, while very powerful, are not potent enough to eliminate all the seeds of karma. Even if it *appears* that our minds and emotions have been totally transformed, the seeds have the ability to germinate given the proper conditions. We may attain those grand heights for a time and then be relegated back to the jurisdiction of the mind and emotions.

When individual consciousness unites with the Divine Conciousness, the illusion of separateness dissolves; this is **Samadhi.**

HIDING ANGER IN A CAVE

There is a wonderful story of a woman who was burdened with a terrible temper. Everything ignited this anger. To control this problem, she decided to retreat into a cave for deep spiritual practice. After spending ten years without seeing another human being, she was convinced the anger had been conquered.

When she finally emerged from the cave and was about to once again enter the world, a crowd gathered, drawn by her vibrant spiritual power. They had known her before and were curious to observe the change.

"What was it like?" one person in the crowd asked. "Did you get angry at all?" said another. "For the entire time, not once did I get angry," she proudly reported.

"It is difficult for me to believe that with the degree of anger you had when you went in, you did not get angry even once," a woman chided.

"No, not even *once*." The cave dweller kept to her story.

"Do you mean, that even if a wild animal came up to your cave and disturbed your meditation, you did not get angry? I really cannot accept what you say as truth," the same woman continued to pursue the issue.

"Listen, *you fool,* I told you, NOTHING DISTURBED MY PEACE AND I NEVER GOT ANGRY. Now leave me alone!"

If the seeds are still fertile, they are always available to sprout. In the deeper states of *Samadhi,* consciousness forever rests in unity with the Divine; then not even a seed is left to germinate.

When one exists in this exalted state, all former identities— woman, man, doctor, nurse, mother, father, Jewish, Christian, Hindu, Muslim—dissolve into oneness. While we still care for and appreciate the body, mind, and emotions as vehicles for living in this physical world, our identification with them lessens. We then may lose interest in anything to do with the physical world, including food, clothing, shelter, and even our relationships. Only a hairs-breadth thread tethers us to our earthly existence.

Our identity has merged with our Divine nature, the all-pervading light within. *Samadhi,* as described by the saints and sages, is a completely different realm of reality than that of our everyday experiences.

We are often inspired by the consciousness brought forth in *Samadhi* to serve the world from that rich understanding. Once we have been ignited by Divine Consciousness, our view of service is forever transformed. With purity of heart and mind, our spiritual vibrations travel through an infinite distance, infusing peace to thousands. We act now out of the knowledge of oneness.

Whichever level of *Samadhi* is experienced, our previous way of understanding life is forever changed. Once we embrace the Divine, our memory clears, as we know who we are without doubt or question. We have fallen in love with our *Divine Self.*

When individual consciousness unites with the Divine Consciousness, the illusion of separateness dissolves; this is Samadhi.

EXPERIENCING THE FLOW OF *DHARANA* (CONTEMPLATION), *DHYANA* (MEDITATION), AND *SAMADHI* (UNION WITH DIVINE CONSCIOUSNESS)

(Please note: This experience is presented to help clarify the evolution and relationship of *Dharana* [contemplation]; *Dhyana* [meditation], and *Samadhi* [Union with Divine Consciousness]. As mentioned earlier, these are not practices in themselves; rather, they are progressive internal "states" that evolve through the influence of conscious living and the other practices, which preceded them. If these states are "invoked" by transforming the effort of "doing" into the natural ease of "being," grace is bestowed.)

Assume a comfortable and relaxed sitting position. Have the base of the spine directed toward the earth, while the top of the head reaches in the direction of the heavens.

Choose an inspirational object for Dharana *(contemplation), something or someone your heart embraces. It could be your sweetheart, child, parent, or friend, or anything that embodies the essence of Divinity for you, such as a statue, picture, or photo. It is effective as long as it uplifts you and allows for an all-encompassing pathway to love.*

Begin to inwardly or outwardly observe all the qualities your senses can elicit.

What are you seeing? Beauty, grace, colors, tones, shapes?

What are you touching? Is it soft, smooth, rounded, sensual, solid?

What are you hearing? Is it gentle, strong, inviting, mesmerizing?

What fragrance is enticing you? Is it sweet, fresh, feminine, masculine, flowery, celestial?

Is your sense of taste involved, perhaps with a kiss?

When you feel the presence of the object of devotion, are you peaceful, happy, joyous, loving?

Allow the physical eyes to close and begin to cuddle up to all the sensory experiences now residing deep within your mind and heart. Embrace the person or the Divine object completely as you encircle it with a feeling of infinite love.

This experience will escort you to the state of Dharana (contemplation).

If your heart forgets to embrace your beloved within, notice how your consciousness wanders away. At these times refresh your thoughts and feelings by either gazing outward or by reforming a clear image within, involving all the senses.

The state of Dharana (contemplation) holds only as long as you can stay present.

After a period of time (minutes, hours, days, weeks, maybe months or longer), the individual sensory perceptions begin to fade and become less defined. Then the identification with the object and its qualities recedes, and simultaneously a deep feeling of love emerges.

Dharana (contemplation) has merged into Dhyana (meditation).

With the immersion into Dhyana (meditation), the cherished object reveals its essence: all-embracing love. With the unveiling of this knowledge, the indrawn focus becomes effortless.

Continue to dwell at this level of Dhyana (meditation) as the all-embracing love flourishes in your heart.

Now, the threshold into Samadhi (Union with Divine Consciousness) is easily traversed. Any remaining thoughts, feelings, and sensory perceptions of the external dissolve. Abounding love is your only experience.

With the immersion into Samadhi, *your entire reality transforms. You experience this all-embracing love for everyone and everything.*

III.4 *When* Dharana *(contemplation),* Dhyana *(meditation), and* Samadhi *(Union with Divine Consciousness) seamlessly merge into one another, this is* Samyama *(fusion).*

III.5 *Through* Samyama, *individual and Divine Consciousness gracefully reunite.*

Samyama (fusion) is the integration of *Dharana, Dhyana,* and *Samadhi. Samyama* starts with *Dharana* (contemplation), focusing on an objective. Here there is an awareness of an object separate from yourself. *Dharana* gracefully slides into *Dhyana* (meditation), when there is an unbroken flow of awareness, allowing identification with the Divine essence of all things. Becoming completely immersed in that essence, individual *consciousness* merges with Divine Consciousness in *Samadhi* (Union with Divine Consciousness).

In *Samyama* (fusion) the three aspects are not perceived as individual but as a single current flowing from uninterrupted awareness. This flow is seamless and without effort. Any effort immediately brings us back into the realm of thoughts and emotions. The ability to realize *Samyama* (fusion) may take years of devoted practice and purification.

Samyama is available in all aspects of life. From the spiritual to the scientific worlds, many great discoveries came through *Samyama*.

We can reflect on the story of the great Albert Einstein that we spoke about in Sutra I. 43, when he experienced *Samadhi* on light. First he contemplated (*Dharana*) light, and with further awareness he was led into meditation (*Dhyana*) on light. These stages followed each other sequentially and united in *Samadhi*. With seamless merging, the experience became *Samyama*.

Einstein humbly proclaimed, "I did not discover light, I meditated on it *[Dhyana]*, until it revealed itself to me *[Samadhi]*."

Through *Samyama* consciousness is reunited. We are now able to realize the essence of Yoga: *Yogah Chitta Vritti Nirodaha. Yoga is the uniting of consciousness in the heart.*

When Dharana (*contemplation*), **Dhyana** (*meditation*), *and* **Samadhi** (*Union with Divine Consciousness*) *seamlessly merge into one another, this is* **Samyama** (*fusion*).

Through Samyama, *individual and Divine Consciousness gracefully reunite.*

EXPERIENCING *SAMYAMA* (FUSION)

When the experience described in Book III, Chapter 1, Sutra 3 (Samadhi, page 261) allows consciousness to gracefully flow from Dharana *continuously to* Dhyana *and into* Samadhi *with burgeoning joy, the experience of* Samyama *(fusion) is fulfilled.*

SUMMARY OF THE REMAINING SUTRAS IN BOOK 111: *Vibhuti Pada*

THE REMAINING SUTRAS in Book III, "*Vibhuti Pada:* The Divine Manifestation of Power," describe the psychic and spiritual powers *(siddhis)* that are the fruits of spiritual practice and *Samyama* (fusion). Although the attainment of these powers *(siddhis)* can be a way of evaluating spiritual progress, we are well and strongly advised not to dwell on them, as they delay us from the ultimate realization of the Divine Self.

There is a wonderful story that helps to explain why certain teachings of Buddha are expounded upon while others are not.

One day while traveling, the Buddha picked up a handful of *simsapa* leaves and asked his disciples what they thought was more numerous: these few leaves he held in his in hand or all the leaves on the trees in the *simsapa* grove.

"Venerable Sir, the *simsapa* leaves that the Blessed One has in his hand are few, but those on all the trees in the *simsapa* grove are more numerous."

"So, too, my disciples, the things I have taught you are few. And why have I not taught so many things?"

The disciples had no answer. So the Buddha replied to his own question with a jewel of spiritual life. "Because they are not as beneficial and relevant to the fundamentals of the holy life, and do not lead to peace, to direct knowledge, to enlightenment, or to Nirvana."

Here are a few examples of the powers described in Book III:

III.24 *By* Samyama *on friendliness, the power to transmit that quality is obtained.*

(This is a sweet one.)

III.25 *By* Samyama *on the strength of elephants, we obtain that level of strength.*

III.26 *By* Samyama *on the Inner Light, one obtains knowledge of what is subtle, hidden, or far distant.*

III.27 *By* Samyama *on the sun, knowledge of the entire solar system is given.*

III.28 *By* Samyama *on the moon comes knowledge of the stars and galaxies.*

III.35 *By* Samyama *on the heart, knowledge of the mind is obtained.*

(The heart as the pathway to the mind.)

III.35 *Through* Samyama *on the heart, awareness of Divine Consciousness dawns.*

(My personal favorite!)

If you venture regularly into the *subtler* aspects of Yoga, the psychic powers are certain to beckon to you. While they can be entertaining and interesting, they are not worth our complete dedication since they distract from the superior illumination and peace beyond their horizons. They may initially excite us, because we have not encountered them before. We would be just as amazed seeing TV for the first time—all those little people moving about in that tiny box. In that way the ordinary mind becomes dazzled by the display of yogic powers. The yogi in her or his equanimity recognizes all these powers as natural aspects of her or his expanded mind and emotions. If they are naturally revealed to you, use this precious gift for the greater good.

These experiences may visit us during our formal practices or at any other time. We may see flashing lights or angels, hear the phone before it rings, choose the scenic road only to find out later that the main highway had been closed for repair, smell blossoms in the winter, or in any number of ways encounter the extraordinary.

Often a disciple may be enticed by these powers (*siddhis*). It is then the role of a guru or spiritual teacher to guide and keep the disciple out of harm's way.

This is the story of one disciple's experience: The long-awaited day of her annual interview with the guru caused her to become very excited. Each year since she came to the ashram, the teacher asked the same question, "How are you progressing with your meditation?" The disciple each time had no choice but to give the same answer. "I am not able to focus my mind and heart for even one moment."

But this time she had some wonderful experiences to share.

She began by telling the guru about the bright lights shooting from the base of her spine, often accompanied by loud chiming sounds. She watched as her beloved teacher carefully listened to her extolling her experiences. As the disciple waited with bated breath to be praised and told how she was *finally* accelerating rapidly in her spiritual growth, the clever guru did the unexpected. Leaning over, the sage touched her on the top of her head, uttering the words, "Don't worry, this will never happen again." *And it never did*.

As the wise Parmahansa Yogananada said, "Meditation is not a circus. Do not be caught by the bright lights and sounds."

Allow yourself to be totally dedicated to the ultimate realization: the knowledge of your Divine Self.

BOOK IV.

KAIVALYA PADA:

Supreme Liberation, A Summary

Book IV, "Kaivalya Pada: *Supreme Liberation*" begins by
further expounding on the attributes of the psychic and
spiritual powers (siddhis). It goes on to emphasize how it
is necessary to transcend the gunas (attributes of nature)
in order to attain liberation, and it proclaims the path of
renunciation as the force that propels the yogi toward
knowing the freedom of her or his own soul.

Book IV then plunges into a valiant attempt to describe
our indescribable cosmic nature, which is beyond qualities
or conditions. Expanding into new dimensions, our consciousness recognizes itself as a limitless and infinite spirit.
Then the exalted yogi radiates supreme wisdom, becoming
a shining beacon of light living only to serve humanity. All
the while, s/he maintains the wisdom and radiance of
the Divine Self.

These passages from the *Bhagavad-Gita* poetically provide a
description of such an illumined yogi:

"What is night for all beings is day for the illumined yogi, resting only in the vision of the Divine Soul."

"When all beings are active with worldly pleasures, the yogi considers this night by keeping herself separate from worldly thoughts, feelings, and ideas."

"Just as waters flow into the ocean, yet the level of the ocean never changes nor is affected by it, similarly one who is steadfast in the Divine Self and by the Divine Self attains liberation."

THE *MAHA VAKYAS* (THE DIVINE EXPRESSIONS)

The earliest seers *(Rishis)* directly experienced and distilled the essential wisdom of the ancient *Vedas* and *Upanishads* into four Divine Expressions, the *Maha Vakyas*. Then the goddess of speech, Vak, leapt from their tongues in all her compassionate splendor, birthing this wisdom to all creation.

This distillation is similar to the way the cow contentedly offers us her sweet milk. All day, she consumes simple grass, and relaxing, she ingests what is suitable to produce the enjoyable beverage and carefully discards the rest. Delighted by the results, we drink her milk and process or culture the rest into other products, including curds, yogurt, cheese, and cream. Cream is churned into butter. For further refinement, the butter is heated to remove the milk solids, leaving only the pure essence of clarified butter, ghee.

The *Rishis* gathered the essence of the Sacred Texts like grass from the subtle realms, refined them, and offered this wisdom, clear and pure as ghee, as the *Maha Vakyas*. This wisdom forms the seeds from which sprout all of the scriptures.

The essence of the timeless *Yogic Scriptures,* when succinctly expressed by the *Maha Vakyas,* allows the heart to know what the mind cannot understand. Through the wisdom of these noble expressions we are able to perceive the essence of all the scriptures.

Each of the *Maha Vakyas* holds the essence from one *Veda* and one *Upanishad.* *Tat Twam Asi* (Thou Art That) is the essential one to comprehend, for it gives rise to the knowledge inherent in the other three. *Tat* (Thou) refers to pure consciousness; *Twam* (That) refers to the reflected consciousness in the individual self; *Asi* (Art, from the verb "to be") proclaims their unity.

Therefore, the statement "Thou Art That" conveys a transcendental experience of oneness that is beyond the body, mind, ego, senses, and sensations.

Reflecting and meditating on the *Maha Vakyas* becomes the bridge that unites us with the Supreme Consciousness. With this realization of the oneness with the Divine, you will *always* remember that you are a Divine Being.

The *Maha Vakyas* (The Divine Expressions)
    Prajnanam Brahma (The cosmic reality is absolute consciousness.)
    The essence of the *Rig Veda* and the *Aitareya Upanishad*

    Tat Twam Asi (Thou Art That)
    The essence of the *Sam Veda* and the *Chandogya Upanishad*

    Ayam Atma Brahma (The individual self and the cosmic Self are one.)
    The essence of the *Atharva Veda* and the *Mandukya Upanishad*

    Aham Brahmasmi (All is that Supreme Consciousness.)
    The essence of the *Yajur Veda* and the *Brihadaranyaka Upanishad*

CONTINUING OUR LIFELONG STUDY
OF THE YOGA SUTRAS

Having journeyed together through the *Yoga Sutras,* we now recognize Yoga as an essential *experiential wisdom* rather than a set of practices or a philosophy. With continued practice and experience, this extremely potent wisdom directs us like a compass to our magnetic Divine nature.

Our wisdom compass has now brought us not just full circle but in an upward spiral, enabling us to revisit the foundational wisdom of the *Yoga Sutras* with a whole new understanding and insight. Each time we begin the study of the *Yoga Sutras* anew, we understand more profoundly—with our hearts—the ever-powerful wisdom they impart.

I myself delved yet again into the sutras to write this book, so that I could express them genuinely from my heart. This process required of me a great deal of faith and devotion. I would recall the many years of sitting with my guru, Sri Swami Satchidanandaji, as he expounded on the meaning of the sutras. I prayed often to the spirits of the goddesses, gods, gurus, saints, and sages to be elevated to Golden Age consciousness and understanding. Many graciously obliged my prayers. But amazingly, it was Sri Patanjali himself, the sage who first compiled the *Yoga Sutras,* who boosted me into a deeper realm of wisdom.

Moving about one of the great temples in South India, paying homage to the many resident goddesses and gods, I was drawn to a small shrine dedicated to "The perfect servant of the Divine," Sri Hanuman, housed in a far-removed area of the temple. Meditating at this shrine, I lost awareness of the physical realm.

Returning to the material plane, I followed the usual custom of circumambulating the shrine. My companions walked at a normal pace; I lagged behind them slightly.

Rounding the final corner of the shrine, I noticed that the sides of the temple were void of decoration or representation. I felt a "wall of energy" that seemed to physically halt me.

At once an "energy vortex" emanating from the blank stone wall drew me to it. When my eyes were able to focus, I saw a tiny oil lamp glowing behind a small, unmarked, soot-covered glass door.

By then my husband and friends had noticed that I was not with them, and they came back to find me, accompanied by a local priest. They seemed not to notice the "energy wall."

"That," said the priest to me, gesturing to the small shrine, "is the *Maha Samadhi* Shrine of Sri Patanjali, the final resting place of his remains."

I stayed transfixed on the spot, and my breathing ceased. After having meditated on what Sri Patanjali could have said, thought, and meant for so many years, he had called me to him, bestowing the blessings of a Divine Being known as *darshan*.

What profound and direct message was he imparting to me? What essence of the *Yoga Sutras* did he divulge to me without spoken words? This will remain a mystery, a deep secret, only known by my heart. I am grateful to have been blessed by Sri Patanjali and the countless others in a multitude of ways, and I pray that what I have expressed in this book reflects the truth of that blessed sanction.

For most of you, the study of Yoga will probably not extend to a pilgrimage to India, or to a lengthy period of study with a realized guru. But if you take what you have experienced in your Yoga practice and bring it into your life, you will find your life greatly improves.

Read the sutras; meditate on them; experience their true meaning. If you do this with your heart, you will know newfound enrichment in your Yoga practice, and in everything you do.

May we live in love and joy knowing our own Divine nature.

Nischala Joy Devi

FOR FURTHER REFLECTION:
THE YOGA SUTRAS
HEARTFULLY EXPRESSED

This section is a listing of the sutras without commentary. They can be recited or written at any time, and are especially powerful as a prelude to meditation. Reading the sutras is a meditative practice of its own.

It is beneficial to reflect on the flow of the *Yoga Sutras* and the way each sets the stage for the next, allowing the meaning of all the sutras in Books I and II and the first five sutras in Book III to be understood with the heart. Reciting them as one continuum allows the essence of the sutras to be conveyed and discovered. *Sravana* (listening) is facilitated by first repeating the sutra aloud, then in a whisper, and finally with only the silence of the heart. This repetition in sequence honors the rhythm of the words and leads us to an understanding greater than each one could elicit individually.

Take a moment to draw in a deep breath and, with wholehearted awareness, repeat these sutras as you *listen* to the great teaching reverberating through your body, mind, emotions, and spirit. Allow the wisdom to be imparted. In this way you will access the deeper, more intuitive form of knowing. May you realize the joy that is your birthright.

1.1   With humility (an open heart and mind), we embrace the sacred study of Yoga.

1.2   Yoga is the uniting of consciousness in the heart.

1.3   United in the heart, consciousness is steadied, then we abide in our true nature—joy.

1.4   At other times, we identify with the rays of consciousness, which fluctuate and encourage our perceived suffering.

1.5   Dividing into five, these rays of consciousness polarize as pleasant or unpleasant.

1.6   The rays manifest as knowledge, misunderstanding, imagination, deep sleep, and memory.

1.7   *Knowledge* embraces personal experience, inference, and insights from the wise.

1.8   *Misunderstanding* comes when perception is unclear or tinted.

1.9   *Imagination* is kindled by hearing words, seeing images, or experiencing feelings.

1.10   *Deep sleep* allows us to withdraw from conscious awareness.

1.11   *Memory* is when a previous experience returns to conscious awareness.

1.12   Consciousness is elevated by *Abhyasa* (Devoted Practice) and *Vairagya* (Remembering the Self).

1.13   Devoted Practice, *Abhyasa,* cultivates the unfolding of consciousness.

1.14   *Abhyasa* is nurtured by a sustained, steady rhythm and a dedicated heart.

1.15   With constant Remembrance of the Self, *Vairagya,* all yearnings fade.

1.16   When consciousness unites, it remains clear and
        unaffected by the external changes of nature, the
        gunas. This is the ultimate *Vairagya*.

1.17   By cultivation of *Abhyasa* and *Vairagya*, the intellect
        becomes keen, reasoning is clear, bliss is reflected to
        all, and outward identification unites with the
        Supreme Consciousness.

1.18   With continued awareness, we identify only with the
        pure consciousness residing in the heart.

1.19   Through identification with pure consciousness, the
        physical world can be transcended.

1.20   This identification is enhanced by faith, dynamism,
        intention, reflection, and perception.

1.21   To the dedicated and devoted, the Divine truth is
        revealed.

1.22   Spiritual Consciousness develops in direct proportion
        to one's dedication.

1.23   Boundless love and devotion unite us with the Divine
        Consciousness.

1.24   The Divine Consciousness is self-effulgent like the sun.

1.25   The Divine is the essence of all knowledge, wisdom,
        and love.

1.26   Knowledge, wisdom, and love are the omnipresent
        teachers, in all beings.

1.27   Repeating the sacred sound manifests Divine Con-
        sciousness.

1.28   When expressed with great devotion, the sacred sound
        reveals our Divine nature.

1.29   By faithful repetition, the inner light luminously shines.

1.30   Perception of our true nature is often obscured by
            physical, mental, and emotional imbalances.

1.31   These imbalances can promote restlessness, uneven
            breathing, worry, and loss of hope.

1.32   These imbalances can be prevented from engaging by
            developing loyalty to a sacred practice.

1.33   To preserve openness of heart and calmness of mind,
            nurture these attitudes:

> *Kindness to those who are happy*
>
> *Compassion for those who are less fortunate*
>
> *Honor for those who embody noble qualities*
>
> *Equanimity to those whose actions oppose your values.*

1.34   Slow, easeful exhalations can be used to restore and
            preserve balance.

1.35   Or engage the focus on an inspiring object.

1.36   Or cultivate devotion to the supreme, ever-blissful
            Light within.

1.37   Or receive grace from a great soul, who exudes Divine
            qualities.

1.38   Or reflect on a peaceful feeling from an experience, a
            dream, or deep sleep.

1.39   Or dedicate yourself to anything that elevates and
            embraces your heart.

1.40   Gradually through focused awareness one's knowledge
            extends from the smallest atom to the greatest magni-
            tude.

1.41   As a naturally pure crystal appears to take the color of
            everything around it yet remains unchanged, the
            yogi's heart remains pure and unaffected by its

surroundings while attaining a state of oneness with
all. This is *Samadhi*.

1.42   When awareness merges with a "material" object or
        form, if the *name, quality*, and *knowledge* are perceived,
        this is *Savitarka Samadhi*, or reflective *Samadhi*.

1.43   When awareness merges with a "material" object or
        form, *if knowledge alone* is perceived, this is *Nirvi-
        tarka Samadhi*, or spontaneous *Samadhi*.

1.44   When awareness merges with a "subtle" object or form,
        two different *Samadhis* are present, *Savichara* (per-
        ceiving *name, quality*, and *knowledge*) and *Nirvichara*
        (perceiving *knowledge alone*).

1.45   These states of *Samadhi* have the power to extend
        beyond all the "material" and "subtle" forms and
        objects, to reveal nature in her unmanifested form.

1.46   All the *Samadhis* described thus far have been *Sabija*
        (with seed), which have the ability to germinate,
        returning us to ordinary consciousness.

1.47   In the purity of *Nirvichara Samadhi*, Divine Conscious-
        ness becomes luminescent.

1.48   When consciousness dwells in *absolute true knowledge*
        (*Ritambhara Prajna*), direct spiritual perception
        dawns.

1.49   This *absolute true knowledge* (*Ritambhara Prajna*) is
        totally different from the knowledge gained by per-
        sonal experience, inference, or insights from the wise.

1.50   When experiencing this *absolute true knowledge*
        (*Ritambhara Prajna*), all previous *Samskaras*
        (impressions) are left behind and new ones are
        prevented from sprouting.

1.51   *Nirbija* (seedless) *Samadhi* outshines all impressions
        and manifestations.

11.1   *Kriya Yoga,* or Yoga in Action, embraces:

    Tapas: igniting the purifying flame.

    Swadhaya: sacred study of the Divine through scripture, nature, and introspection.

    Iswara Pranidhana: wholehearted dedication to the Divine Light in all.

11.2   These practices enhance inner awareness and guide us to liberation.

11.3   Dissolving the five *Kleshas,* or veils, brings forth the radiance of the Divine Self.

The five *Kleshas*, or veils, are:

    Avidya: innocence of our Divine nature

    Asmita: undue trust in the individual self

    Raga: excessive fondness of fleeting pleasures

    Dvesa: excessive avoidance of unpleasant experiences

    Abhinivesah: elusive awareness of immortality.

11.4   Innocence of our Divine nature (*Avidya*) creates a fertile field where the dormant seeds of the other four veils take root.

11.5   Innocence of our Divine nature (*Avidya*) encourages identification with the ever changing, rather than with the inner stillness of the heart.

11.6   When undue trust is placed in the individual self (*Asmita*), it is confused with the Divine Self.

11.7   Excessive fondness for fleeting pleasures (*Raga*) causes longing.

11.8   Excessive avoidance of unpleasant experiences (*Dvesa*) causes disdain.

11.9   The elusive awareness of immortality is inherent even
            for the wise (*Abhinivesah*).

11.10   With keen observation and discretion, these *Kleshas*
            become translucent.

11.11   If they have manifested into action, the veils must be
            dissolved through inward practice.

11.12   The womb of karma (*Karmasala*), sheathed by the
            Kleshas (veils), gives birth to experiences now and in
            the future.

11.13   As long as the veils encase the womb of karma
            (*Karmasala*), all actions will be affected.

11.14   Karma bears fruits according to the type and quality of
            the seed planted, and the care given to its growth.

11.15   Intuitive Wisdom empowers us to expand beyond the
            constantly changing natural world (seen) to the
            abode of the Divine Spirit (seer).

11.16   With this understanding, once-vital difficulties become
            impotent.

11.17   The source of these difficulties is the inability to recog-
            nize the Divine Spirit (seer) as omniscient and there-
            fore separate from the constantly changing natural
            world (seen).

11.18   When understood as illusory (*Maya*), nature (seen) and
            her attributes the *gunas* exist to serve the Divine Self
            (seer) with both enjoyment and liberation.

11.19   These attributes of nature (*gunas*) are both tangible and
            intangible.

11.20   The Divine Self (seer) observes the world without being
            affected by it.

11.21   The natural world (seen) exists for benefit of the Divine
            Self (seer).

11.22   With realization of the Divine Self (seer), the illusory natural world (seen) becomes transparent, though still seemingly very real to those enmeshed in it.

11.23   When the Divine Self (seer) and nature (seen) unite, this dynamic and powerful synergy creates the illusory world, obscuring the vision of spirit.

11.24   This union is consummated when we forget the Divine Self (seer).

11.25   With constant remembrance of the Divine Self, no such union is possible.

11.26   Established in the grace of Intuitive Wisdom, we experience liberation.

11.27   Liberation is recognized in seven ways: when we no longer feel the need for knowledge, to stay away from anything or anyone, to gather material things, or to act. Our constant companions are joy, faith, and clarity.

11.28   By embracing *Asthaanga Yoga,* the Eight-Faceted Path, Intuitive Wisdom dawns and reveals our inner radiance.

11.29   Asthaanga Yoga, the Eight-Faceted Path, embraces:

> *Yama:* reflection of our true nature
>
> *Niyama:* evolution toward harmony
>
> *Asana:* comfort in being, posture
>
> *Pranayama:* enhancement and guidance of universal *prana* (energy)
>
> *Pratyahara:* encouraging the senses to draw within
>
> *Dharana:* gathering and focusing of consciousness inward
>
> *Dhyana:* continuous inward flow of consciousness
>
> *Samadhi:* union with Divine Consciousness.

II.30   *Yama* (reflection of our true nature) is experienced through:

> *Ahimsa:* reverence, love, compassion for all.
>
> *Satya:* truthfulness, integrity.
>
> *Astheya:* generosity, honesty
>
> *Brahmacharya:* balance and moderation of the vital life force
>
> *Aparigraha:* awareness of abundance, fulfillment.

II.31   These great truths are universal and inherent to all beings. If altered or ignored, the quality of life is greatly compromised.

II.32   *Niyama* (evolution toward harmony) encompasses:

> *Saucha:* simplicity, purity, refinement
>
> *Santosha:* contentment, being at peace with oneself and others
>
> *Tapas:* igniting the purifying flame
>
> *Swadhaya:* sacred study of the Divine through scripture, nature, and introspection
>
> *Iswara Pranidhana:* wholehearted dedication to the Divine.

II.33   When presented with disquieting thoughts or feelings, cultivate an opposite, elevated attitude, this is *Pratipaksha Bhavana*.

II.34   The desire to act upon unwholesome thoughts or actions or to cause or condone others toward these thoughts or actions is preventable, this is also *Pratipaksha Bhavana*.

II.35   Embracing reverence and love for all (*Ahimsa*), we experience oneness.

II.36   Dedicated to truth and integrity (*Satya*), our thoughts, words, and actions gain the power to manifest.

II.37   Abiding in generosity and honesty (*Astheya*), material and spiritual prosperity is bestowed.

II.38   Dedicated to living a balanced and moderate life (*Brahmacharya*), the scope of one's life force becomes boundless.

II.39   Acknowledging abundance (*Aparigraha*), we recognize the blessings in everything and gain insights into the purpose of our wordly existence.

II.40   Through simplicity and continual refinement (*Saucha*), the body, thoughts, and emotions become clear reflections of the Self within.

II.41   *Saucha* reveals our joyful nature, and the yearning for knowing the Self blossoms.

II.42   When at peace and content with oneself and others (*Santosha*), supreme joy is celebrated.

II.43   Living life with zeal and sincerity, the purifying flame is ignited (*Tapas*), revealing the inner light.

II.44   Sacred study of the Divine through scripture, nature, and introspection (*Swadhaya*) guides us to the Supreme Self.

II.45   Through wholehearted dedication (*Iswara Prandihaha*), we become intoxicated with the Divine.

II.46   The natural comfort and joy of our being is expressed when the body becomes steady (asana).

II.47   As the body yields all efforts and holdings, the infinite within is revealed.

II.48   Thereafter we are freed from the flucuations of the *gunas*.

11.49	The universal life force (*prana*) is enhanced and guided through the harmonious rhythm of the breath (*pranayama*).
11.50	The movement of the life force is influenced by inhalation, exhalation and sustained breath.
11.51	A balanced rhythmical pattern steadies the mind and emotions, causing the breath to become motionless.
11.52	As a result, the veils over the inner light are lifted.
11.53	The vista of higher consciousness is revealed.
11.54	Encouraging the senses to draw inward is *pratyahara*.
11.55	Glimpsing the inner light, the senses contentedly dwell within.
III.1	Gathering consciousness and focusing it within is *Dharana* (contemplation).
III.2	The continuous inward flow of consciousness is *Dhyana* (meditation).
III.3	When individual consciousness unites with the Divine Consciousness, the illusion of separateness dissolves; this is *Samadhi*.
III.4	When *Dharana* (contemplation), *Dhyana* (meditation), *and Samadhi* (union with Divine Consciousness) seamlessly merge into one another; this is *Samyama* (fusion).
III.5	Through *Samyama*, individual and Divine Consciousness gracefully reunite.

ACKNOWLEDGMENTS

With Gratitude

It was the women, so many of them over the years, who encouraged and yes, at times cajoled me to take on this ominous project. My heart wanted to keep my way of seeing the teachings nestled within it. "You have to write this book for us," they told me. Now that it is birthed, my gratitude is wrapped in their eagerness for the sutras representing them, in "their language."

The numerous nameless faces come back to me as I begin to pour out my gratitude, the magnitude of which cannot begin to be expressed. My hope is that in naming a few I will also recognize the others.

I begin with my mother, whose faith in me was unwavering; in her eyes and heart, I could do *anything*. Although being a woman in her lifetime may have hindered *her* way of life, she made sure the prejudices did not funnel my life into small thinking. My father by his example showed me that following your own heart was not always popular, but the only way to live.

With gratitude I honor all my teachers, formal and informal, who brought the scriptures, especially the *Yoga Sutras*, to life for me. Sri Swami Satchidanandaji, whose clear and simple yet profound way of telling them enabled me to absorb them immediately into a new way of living. Mataji Indra Devi and other teachers, who continued to inspire me either through their example or their writings.

To all the students I taught, who experienced the heart of the *Yoga Sutras* and reflected their experiences back to me. Encouraging me, they chanted, "*You* are the one to write this book!"

In the actual writing of the book, Prakasha Shakti contributed her own love and knowledge of the sutras, helping me to explain an often esoteric concept simply. Carol Krukoff, an exceptional writer and friend, lent hand and heart to helping me form these ideas in such a way that the publisher could begin to understand what an extraordinary feat this was. She offered her help, she said, "as a labor of love" for "my daughter and her friends."

For arranging me to "try out" some of these ideas on students, I want to appreciate Robin Rothenberg, who said, "If no one will publish it, I will personally raise the money to do it!" Thanks to Hansa Knox, Patricia Sullivan, Sarah Powers, Robin Gueth, Bhavani Butterfield-Brown, and the continuing support of Janice Gates, who was writing about women and yoga at the same time that I was writing *The Secret Power of Yoga*. To my dear sister-friend Laurel, whose enthusiasm encourages me to dream the possible dream.

This project was infused with much masculine support, from the male students, who wanted another, more heartfelt voice to the sutras, to my soul mate, Bhaskar Deva, who allowed himself to be educated as to the prejudices and inhibition of the feminine power, saying, "That many women were persecuted! I had no idea. This is important; you must add this to the book!" His unwavering love keeps me in my heart.

David Frawley (Pandit Vamadeva Shastri), a great modern-day pundit, encouraged me to "tell the sutras from the heart," affirming to me that *chitta* means heart, not mind. For helping to clarify the more esoteric sutras, I thank Swami Swroopanandaji and my dear friend and Hindu priest, Krishnanambudri.

I had asked the Divine for a great team to help birth this book. My agent, Loretta Barrett, who believed in the project from the start. Shaye Areheart, who as always encouraged me. Julia Pastore, a great and compassionate editor, who at times became my cheerleader. Peter Guzzardi, my "male" editor, who lent his expertise to make the manuscript shine while reflecting the compassionate heart that resides in female and male alike.

The mystical gratitude is less easy to express. While at the computer, surrounded by all the aspects of the feminine Divine I could find, I was constantly playing the Saraswati (goddess of wisdom and knowledge) mantra. The goddess Saraswati (and Vak, goddess of speech) has been my constant companion and spirit writer in this awesome outpouring of love. I know that without Divine grace, this book would not have been possible.

INDEX

</>

NISCHALA JOY DEVI is a master teacher and healer. For more than thirty years she has been highly respected as an international advocate for her innovative way of expressing Yoga and its subtle uses for spiritual growth and complete healing.

She was a monastic student of the world-renowned Yogiraj Sri Swami Satchidananda and spent more than twenty-five years receiving his direct guidance and teachings. During her time in the monastery, she began to blend Western medicine with Yoga and meditation. She then offered her expertise in developing the Yoga portion of the Dean Ornish Program for Reversing Heart Disease, where she subsequently served for seven years as director of Stress Management. She also cofounded the award-winning Commonweal Cancer Help Program.

Nischala Devi produced the "Abundant Well-Being Series" CDs to allow these simple yet profound Yoga and stress-relieving techniques to reach more people. Her book *The Healing Path of Yoga,* now in its sixth printing, also expresses these teachings.

With her knowledge of Yoga and her experience in assisting those with life-threatening diseases, she created *Yoga of the Heart,* a training and certification program for Yoga teachers and health professionals designed to adapt Yoga practices to the special needs of that population.

Nischala Devi is now directing her energies to bringing the feminine heart perspective back into spirituality and the scriptures. When not traveling and teaching, she lives with her husband in northern California and Mexico.

For information on programs, training, and retreats, please visit her website www.abundantwellbeing.com.

Yoga with the Power to Heal

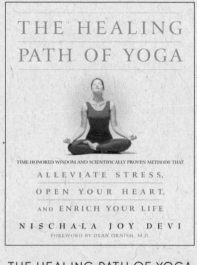

THE HEALING PATH OF YOGA
$17.00 paper ($25.95 Canada) •
978-0-609-80502-2

With visualizations, breathing practices, and meditations, as well as by providing the classic steps and illustrated instructions for yoga's physical poses, *The Healing Path of Yoga* uses timeless evidence-based yoga techniques and philosophy, along with Nischala Joy Devi's lifestyle-altering regimen, to create one extraordinary program with the power to rejuvenate and heal. *The Healing Path of Yoga* presents the key to preventing disease as well as supporting weight loss, relaxation, and overall wellness of body, mind, and spirit.

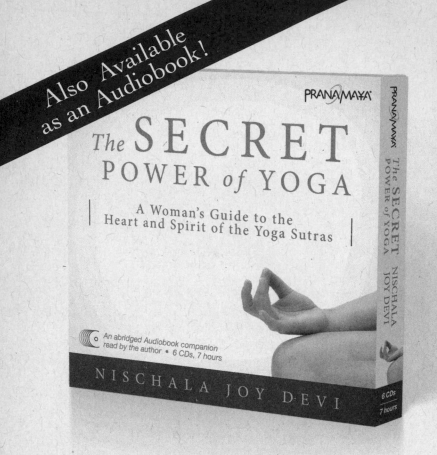